THE PLANT-B... DIET FOR COUPLE

2 BOOKS IN 1

Cookbook

More than **220** High-Protein Vegetarian Recipes **to Surprise your Partner** in the Kitchen! Start your Healthier Lifestyle with the Best Green Meals to **Make Together!**

By

William Miller

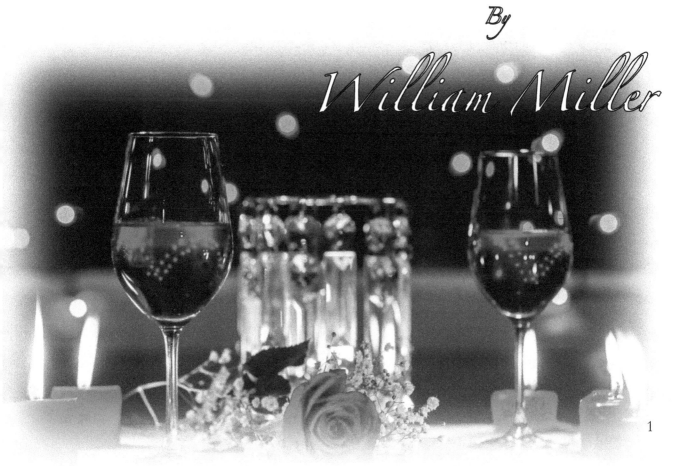

Table of Contents

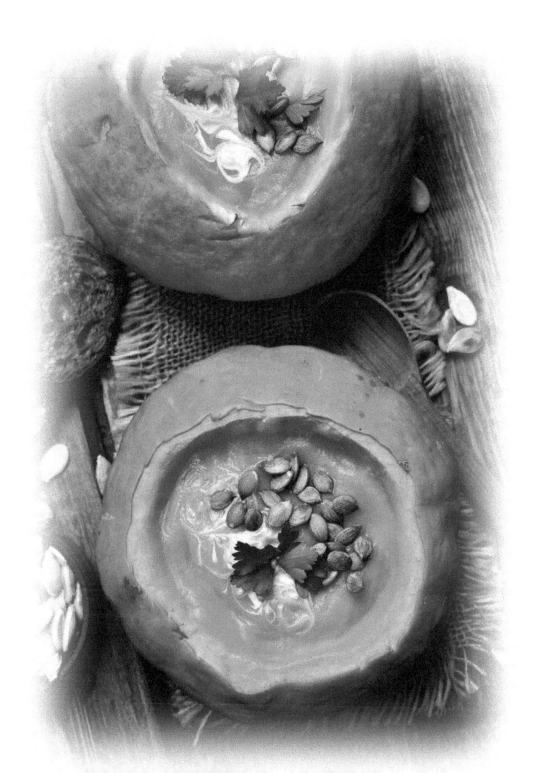

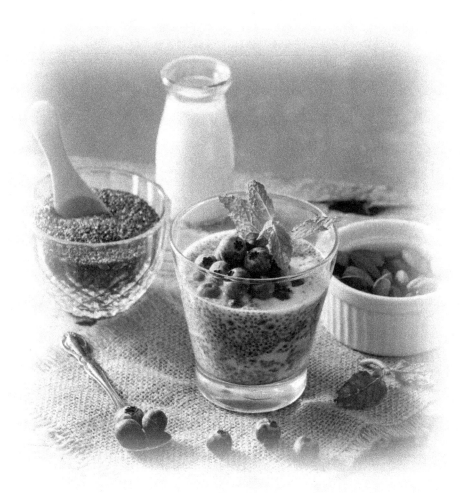

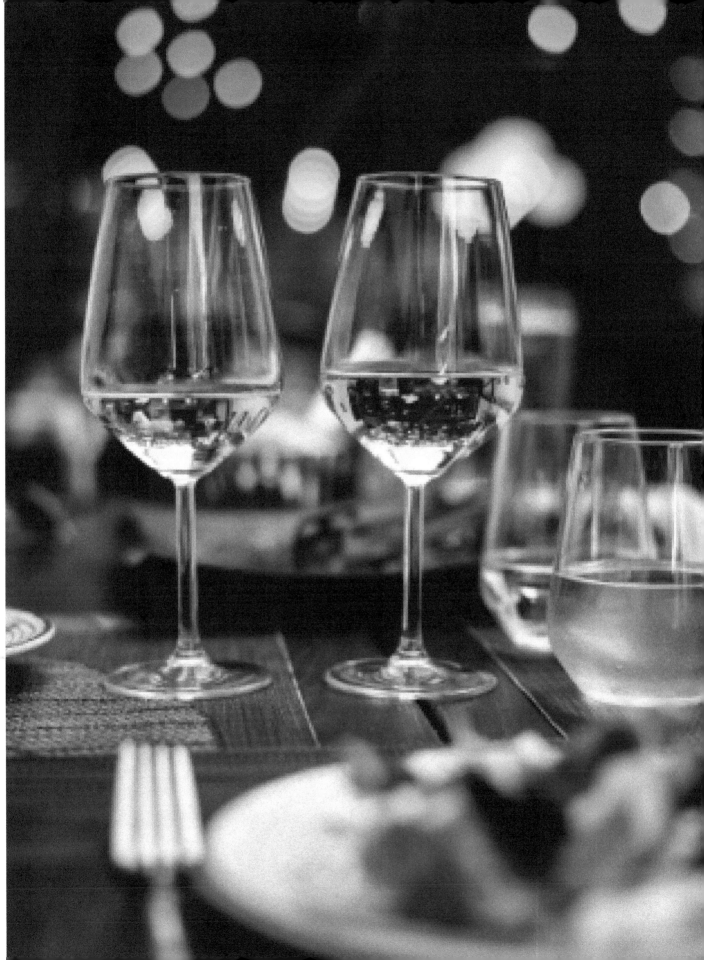

Introduction

Do you know what is good for your body?

Do you know that each family member should eat different portions and different food according to gender, weight and lifestyle?

And, most importantly: do you ever make a list of the foods you eat just to count the junk and tell yourself "it will get better next week?"

Clinical studies show that in ancient times, humans ate mainly harvested foods that grew wild on the ground. This is also evidenced by our teeth: they are more similar to herbivorous animals, which use them to grind nuts or chew herbs for long periods of time, than those of carnivores, which use them to tear and tear meat from the body of their prey.
Thanks to this growing body of information and proven clinical studies, people are increasingly interested in eating less processed foods, and this trend has turned many people into vegetarians or even vegans.

The Plant-Based diet allows you to get the right amount of nutrients and follow an eating plan that makes you light and fit, that's why it's the best solution!

In recent years, people have become increasingly concerned about what they eat.
It is important to eat healthy foods, without preservatives or additives, to provide the right nutrients to the body.
Scientists say to eat natural and minimally processed foods, and in this only one diet meets this need: **the Plant-Based Diet!**

The Plant-Based Diet is based on *fruits*, *vegetables* and *nuts*, without any nutritional intake from animal protein. Eating only plant-based foods your body can work better and can stay LIGHT! A student must feel light and have energy to study well and pass his/her exams!
If you eat meat (especially red meat) or heavy animal proteins, or many carbs, your body feels tired and you feel sleepy! This no happens if you eat plant-based foods!

The Plant-Based diet is suitable for everyone: kids, over 50, athletes, women, men and it's easy to learn even for beginners! This is why I have created a series of books on the Plant-Based diet each specific for each category of people!

However, how many times you went crazy to cook different plates for your partner and you? Too many! I have often listlessly cooked for my partner just because I didn't have bright ideas in my life. So, I decided to create this book to help all couples always find a tasty recipe every day for both of them!
I created this Plant-Based cookbook specific for Couple: this is a collection of 2 of my best books, **"The Plant-Based for MEN Cookbook"** and **"The Plant-Based for WOMEN cookbook"**, to give all my readers more than 220 fantastic recipes!

Are you ready to discover the best Plant-Based recipes? GO!

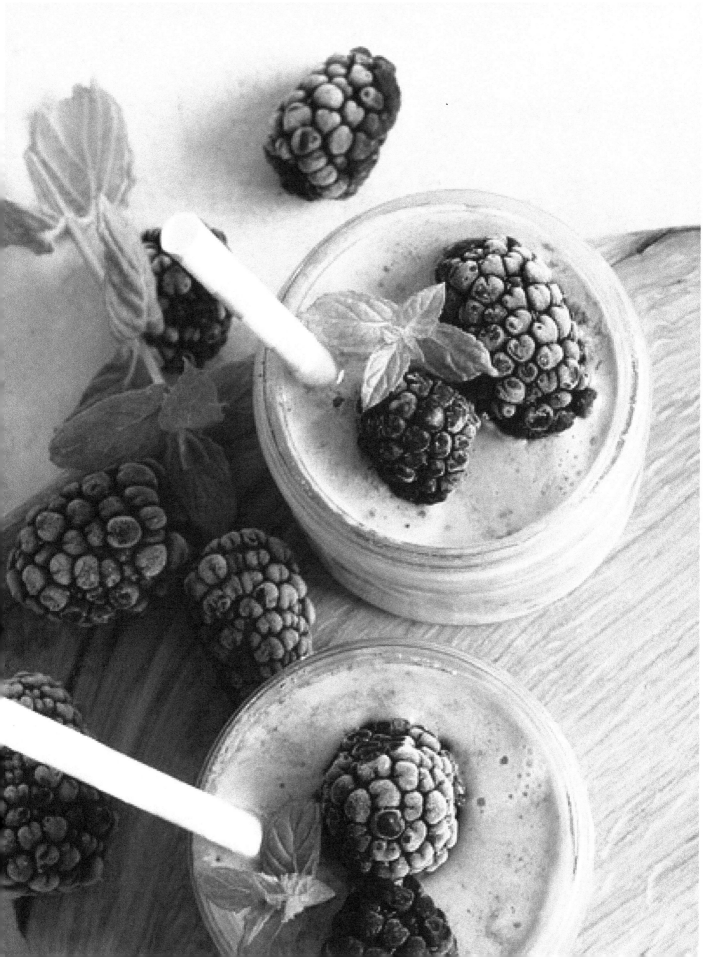

Chapter 1. BREAKFAST AND SNACKS

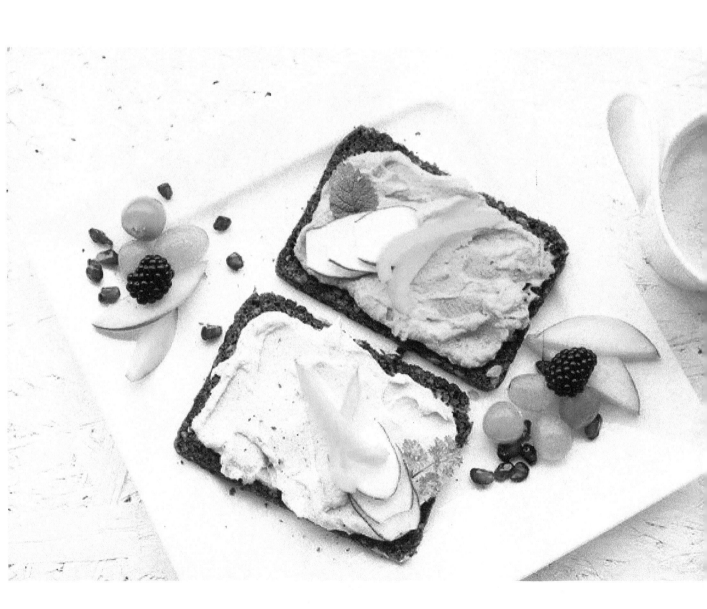

1) FRENCH TOASTS TROPICAL STYLE

Preparation Time: 55 minutes		Servings: 4

Ingredients:

- ✓ 2 tbsp flax seed powder
- ✓ 1 ½ cups unsweetened almond milk
- ✓ ½ cup almond flour
- ✓ 2 tbsp maple syrup + extra for drizzling
- ✓ 2 pinches of salt
- ✓ ½ tbsp cinnamon powder
- ✓ ½ tsp fresh lemon zest
- ✓ 1 tbsp fresh pineapple juice
- ✓ 8 whole-grain bread slices

Directions:

Preheat the oven to 400 F and lightly grease a roasting rack with olive oil. Set aside.

In a medium bowl, mix the flax seed powder with 6 tbsp water and allow thickening for 5 to 10 minutes. Whisk in the almond milk, almond flour, maple syrup, salt, cinnamon powder, lemon zest, and pineapple juice. Soak the bread on both sides in the almond milk mixture and allow sitting on a plate for 2 to 3 minutes.

Heat a large skillet over medium heat and place the bread in the pan. Cook until golden brown on the bottom side. Flip the bread and cook further until golden brown on the other side, 4 minutes in total. Transfer to a plate, drizzle some maple syrup on top and serve immediately

2) SPECIAL CREPES WITH MUSHROOM

Preparation Time: 25 minutes		Servings: 4

Ingredients:

- ✓ 1 cup whole-wheat flour
- ✓ 1 tsp onion powder
- ✓ ½ tsp baking soda
- ✓ ¼ tsp salt
- ✓ 1 cup pressed, crumbled tofu
- ✓ ⅓ cup plant-based milk
- ✓ ¼ cup lemon juice
- ✓ 2 tbsp extra-virgin olive oil
- ✓ ½ cup finely chopped mushrooms
- ✓ ½ cup finely chopped onion
- ✓ 2 cups collard greens

Directions:

Combine the flour, onion powder, baking soda, and salt in a bowl. Blitz the tofu, milk, lemon juice, and oil in a food processor over high speed for 30 seconds. Pour over the flour mixture and mix to combine well. Add in the mushrooms, onion, and collard greens.

Heat a skillet and grease with cooking spray. Lower the heat and spread a ladleful of the batter across the surface of the skillet. Cook for 4 minutes on both sides or until set. Remove to a plate. Repeat the process until no batter is left, greasing with a little more oil, if needed. Serve

3) SPECIAL FRENCH TOAST WITH CINNAMON-BANANA

Preparation Time: 25 minutes		Servings: 3

Ingredients:

- ✓ 1/3 cup coconut milk
- ✓ 1/2 cup banana, mashed
- ✓ 2 tbsp besan (chickpea flour)
- ✓ 1/2 tsp baking powder
- ✓ 1/2 tsp vanilla paste
- ✓ A pinch of sea salt
- ✓ 1 tbsp agave syrup
- ✓ 1/2 tsp ground allspice
- ✓ A pinch of grated nutmeg
- ✓ 6 slices day-old sourdough bread
- ✓ 2 bananas, sliced
- ✓ 2 tbsp brown sugar
- ✓ 1 tsp ground cinnamon

Directions:

To make the batter, thoroughly combine the coconut milk, mashed banana, besan, baking powder, vanilla, salt, agave syrup, allspice and nutmeg.

Dredge each slice of bread into the batter until well coated on all sides.

Preheat an electric griddle to medium heat and lightly oil it with a nonstick cooking spray.

Cook each slice of bread on the preheated griddle for about 3 minutes per side until golden brown.

Garnish the French toast with the bananas, brown sugar and cinnamon. Enjoy

4) INDIAN AUTHENTIC ROTI

Preparation Time: 30 minutes		Servings: 5

Ingredients:

- ✓ 2 cups bread flour
- ✓ 1 tsp baking powder
- ✓ 1/2 tsp salt
- ✓ 3/4 warm water
- ✓ 1 cup vegetable oil, for frying

Directions:

Thoroughly combine the flour, baking powder and salt in a mixing bowl. Gradually add in the water until the dough comes together.

Divide the dough into five balls; flatten each ball to create circles.

Heat the olive oil in a frying pan over a moderately high flame. Fry the first bread, turning it over to promote even cooking; fry it for about 10 minutes or until golden brown.

Repeat with the remaining dough. Transfer each roti to a paper towel-lined plate to drain the excess oil.

Enjoy

5) TYPICAL CHIA CHOCOLATE PUDDING

Preparation Time: 10 minutes + chilling time		Servings: 4

Ingredients:

- ✓ 4 tbsp unsweetened cocoa powder
- ✓ 4 tbsp maple syrup
- ✓ 1 2/3 cups coconut milk
- ✓ A pinch of grated nutmeg
- ✓ A pinch of ground cloves
- ✓ 1/2 tsp ground cinnamon
- ✓ 1/2 cup chia seeds

Directions:

Add the cocoa powder, maple syrup, milk and spices to a bowl and stir until everything is well incorporated.

Add in the chia seeds and stir again to combine well. Spoon the mixture into four jars, cover and place in your refrigerator overnight.

On the actual day, stir with a spoon and serve. Enjoy

6) QUICK BREAKFAST POLENTA

Preparation Time: 20 minutes		Servings: 2

Ingredients:

- ✓ 2 cups vegetable broth
- ✓ 1/2 cup cornmeal
- ✓ 1/2 tsp sea salt
- ✓ 1/4 tsp ground black pepper, to taste
- ✓ 1/4 tsp red pepper flakes, crushed
- ✓ 2 tbsp olive oil

Directions:

In a medium saucepan, bring the vegetable broth to boil over medium-high heat. Now, add in the cornmeal, whisking continuously to prevent lumps.

Season with salt, black pepper and red pepper.

Reduce the heat to a simmer. Continue to simmer, whisking periodically, for about 18 minutes, until the mixture has thickened.

Now, pour the olive oil into a saucepan and stir to combine well. Enjoy

7) EASY PEPPER AND SCALLION OMELETTE

Preparation Time: 15 minutes		Servings: 2

Ingredients:

- ✓ 2 tbsp olive oil
- ✓ 3 scallions, chopped
- ✓ 2 bell peppers, chopped
- ✓ 6 tbsp besan (chickpea flour)
- ✓ 10 tbsp rice milk, unsweetened
- ✓ Kala namak salt and ground black pepper, to season
- ✓ 1/3 tsp red pepper flakes
- ✓ 2 tbsp fresh Italian parsley, chopped

Directions:

Heat the olive oil in a frying pan over medium-high heat. Once hot, sauté the scallions and peppers for about 3 minutes until tender and aromatic.

Meanwhile, whisk the chickpea flour with the milk, salt, black pepper and red pepper flakes.

Then, pour the mixture into the frying pan.

Cook for about 4 minutes. Turn it over and cook for an additional 3 to 4 minutes until set. Serve with fresh parsley. Enjoy

8) ORIGINAL TOFU SCRAMBLE

Preparation Time: 15 minutes		Servings: 2

Ingredients:

- ✓ 1 tbsp olive oil
- ✓ 6 ounces extra-firm tofu, pressed and crumbled
- ✓ 1 cup baby spinach
- ✓ Sea salt and ground black pepper to taste
- ✓ 1/2 tsp turmeric powder
- ✓ 1/4 tsp cumin powder
- ✓ 1/2 tsp garlic powder
- ✓ 1 handful fresh chives, chopped

Directions:

Heat the olive oil in a frying skillet over medium heat. When it's hot, add the tofu and sauté for 8 minutes, stirring occasionally to promote even cooking.

Add in the baby spinach and aromatics and continue sautéing an additional 1 to 2 minutes.

Garnish with fresh chives and serve warm. Enjoy

9) SPECIAL FRENCH TOAST WITH BANANA AND STRAWBERRY SYRUP

Preparation Time: 40 minutes		Servings: 8

Ingredients:

- ✓ 1 banana, mashed
- ✓ 1 cup coconut milk
- ✓ 1 tsp pure vanilla extract
- ✓ ¼ tsp ground nutmeg
- ✓ ½ tsp ground cinnamon
- ✓ 1 ½ tsp arrowroot powder
- ✓ A pinch of salt
- ✓ 8 slices whole-grain bread
- ✓ 1 cup strawberries
- ✓ 2 tbsp water
- ✓ 2 tbsp maple syrup

Directions:

Preheat oven to 350 F.

In a bowl, stir banana, coconut milk, vanilla, nutmeg, cinnamon, arrowroot, and salt. Dip each bread slice in the banana mixture and arrange on a baking tray. Spread the remaining banana mixture over the top. Bake for 30 minutes until the tops are lightly browned. In a pot over medium heat, put the strawberries, water, and maple syrup. Simmer for 15-10 minutes, until the berries breaking up and the liquid has reduced. Serve

10) LOVELY PIMIENTO BISCUITS WITH CASHEW CHEESE

Preparation Time: 30 minutes		Servings: 4

Ingredients:

- ✓ 2 cups whole-wheat flour
- ✓ 2 tsp baking powder
- ✓ 1 tsp salt
- ✓ ½ tsp baking soda
- ✓ ½ tsp garlic powder
- ✓ ¼ tsp black pepper
- ✓ ¼ cup plant butter, cold and cubed
- ✓ ¾ cup coconut milk
- ✓ 1 cup shredded cashew cheese
- ✓ 1 (4 oz) jar chopped pimientos,
- ✓ 1 tbsp melted unsalted plant butter

Directions:

Preheat the oven to 450 F and line a baking sheet with parchment paper. Set aside. In a medium bowl, mix the flour, baking powder, salt, baking soda, garlic powder, and black pepper. Add the cold butter using a hand mixer until the mixture is the size of small peas. Pour in ¾ of the coconut milk and continue whisking. Continue adding the remaining coconut milk, a tbspful at a time, until dough forms.

Mix in the cashew cheese and pimientos. (If the dough is too wet to handle, mix in a little bit more flour until it is manageable). Place the dough on a lightly floured surface and flatten the dough into ½-inch thickness.

Use a 2 ½-inch round cutter to cut out biscuits' pieces from the dough. Gather, re-roll the dough once and continue cutting out biscuits. Arrange the biscuits on the prepared pan and brush the tops with the melted butter.

Bake for 12-14 minutes, or until the biscuits are golden brown. Cool and serve

11) SWEET RASPBERRY, ORANGE-GLAZED MUFFINS

Preparation Time: 40 minutes		Servings: 4

Ingredients:

- ✓ 2 tbsp flax seed powder
- ✓ 2 cups whole-wheat flour
- ✓ 1 ½ tsp baking powder
- ✓ A pinch salt
- ✓ ½ cup plant butter, softened
- ✓ 2 cups pure date sugar
- ✓ ½ cup oat milk
- ✓ 2 tsp vanilla extract
- ✓ 1 lemon, zested
- ✓ 1 cup dried raspberries
- ✓ 2 tbsp orange juice

Directions:

Preheat oven to 400 F and grease 6 muffin cups with cooking spray. In a small bowl, mix the flax seed powder with 6 tbsp water and allow thickening for 5 minutes to make the vegan "flax egg." In a medium bowl, mix the flour, baking powder, and salt. In another bowl, cream the plant butter, half of the date sugar, and vegan "flax egg." Mix in the oat milk, vanilla, and lemon zest.

Combine both mixtures, fold in raspberries, and fill muffin cups two-thirds way up with the batter. Bake for 20-25 minutes. In a medium bowl, whisk orange juice and remaining date sugar until smooth. Remove the muffins when ready and transfer to a wire rack to cool. Drizzle the glaze on top to serve

12) RED STRAWBERRY AND PECAN BREAKFAST

Preparation Time: 15 minutes		Servings: 2

Ingredients:

- ✓ 1 (14-oz) can coconut milk, refrigerated overnight
- ✓ 1 cup granola
- ✓ ½ cup pecans, chopped
- ✓ 1 cup sliced strawberries

Directions:

- • Drain the coconut milk liquid. Layer the coconut milk solids, granola, and strawberries in small glasses. Top with chopped pecans and serve right away

13) TASTY GRANOLA WITH HAZELNUTS AND ORANGE

Preparation Time: 50 minutes		Servings: 5

Ingredients:

- ✓ 2 cups rolled oats
- ✓ ¾ cup whole-wheat flour
- ✓ 1 tbsp ground cinnamon
- ✓ 1 tsp ground ginger
- ✓ ½ cup sunflower seeds

- ✓ ½ cup hazelnuts, chopped
- ✓ ½ cup pumpkin seeds
- ✓ ½ cup shredded coconut
- ✓ 1 ¼ cups orange juice
- ✓ ½ cup dried cherries
- ✓ ½ cup goji berries

Directions:

Preheat oven to 350 F.

In a bowl, combine the oats, flour, cinnamon, ginger, sunflower seeds, hazelnuts, pumpkin seeds, and coconut. Pour in the orange juice, toss to mix well.

Transfer to a baking sheet and bake for 15 minutes. Turn the granola and continue baking until it is crunchy, about 30 minutes. Stir in the cherries and goji berries and store in the fridge for up to 14 days

14) SIMPLE ORANGE CREPES

Preparation Time: 30 minutes		Servings: 4

Ingredients:

- ✓ 2 tbsp flax seed powder
- ✓ 1 tsp vanilla extract
- ✓ 1 tsp pure date sugar
- ✓ ¼ tsp salt

- ✓ 2 cups almond flour
- ✓ 1 ½ cups oat milk
- ✓ ½ cup melted plant butter
- ✓ 3 tbsp fresh orange juice
- ✓ 3 tbsp plant butter for frying

Directions:

In a medium bowl, mix the flax seed powder with 6 tbsp water and allow thickening for 5 minutes to make the vegan "flax egg." Whisk in the vanilla, date sugar, and salt.

Pour in a quarter cup of almond flour and whisk, then a quarter cup of oat milk, and mix until no lumps remain. Repeat the mixing process with the remaining almond flour and almond milk in the same quantities until exhausted.

Mix in the plant butter, orange juice, and half of the water until the mixture is runny like pancakes. Add the remaining water until the mixture is lighter. Brush a non-stick skillet with some butter and place over medium heat to melt.

Pour 1 tbsp of the batter into the pan and swirl the skillet quickly and all around to coat the pan with the batter. Cook until the batter is dry and golden brown beneath, about 30 seconds.

Use a spatula to flip the crepe and cook the other side until golden brown too. Fold the crepe onto a plate and set aside. Repeat making more crepes with the remaining batter until exhausted. Drizzle some maple syrup on the crepes and serve

15) ENGLISH OAT BREAD WITH COCONUT

Preparation Time: 50 minutes		Servings: 4

Ingredients:

- ✓ 4 cups whole-wheat flour
- ✓ ¼ tsp salt
- ✓ ½ cup rolled oats

- ✓ 1 tsp baking soda
- ✓ 1 ¾ cups coconut milk, thick
- ✓ 2 tbsp pure maple syrup

Directions:

Preheat the oven to 400 F.

In a bowl, mix flour, salt, oats, and baking soda. Add in coconut milk and maple syrup and whisk until dough forms. Dust your hands with some flour and knead the dough into a ball. Shape the dough into a circle and place on a baking sheet.

Cut a deep cross on the dough and bake in the oven for 15 minutes at 450 F. Reduce the temperature to 400 F and bake further for 20 to 25 minutes or until a hollow sound is made when the bottom of the bread is tapped. Slice and serve

17

16) MEXICAN BOWL WITH BLACK BEANS AND SPICY QUINOA

Preparation Time: 25 minutes		Servings: 4

Ingredients:

- ✓ 1 cup brown quinoa, rinsed
- ✓ 3 tbsp plant-based yogurt
- ✓ ½ lime, juiced
- ✓ 2 tbsp chopped fresh cilantro
- ✓ 1 (5 oz) can black beans, drained
- ✓ 3 tbsp tomato salsa
- ✓ ¼ avocado, sliced
- ✓ 2 radishes, shredded
- ✓ 1 tbsp pepitas (pumpkin seeds)

Directions:

Cook the quinoa with 2 cups of slightly salted water in a medium pot over medium heat or until the liquid absorbs, 15 minutes. Spoon the quinoa into serving bowls and fluff with a fork.

In a small bowl, mix the yogurt, lime juice, cilantro, and salt. Divide this mixture on the quinoa and top with the beans, salsa, avocado, radishes, and pepitas. Serve immediately

17) ITALIAN ALMOND AND RAISIN GRANOLA

Preparation Time: 20 minutes		Servings: 8

Ingredients:

- ✓ 5 ½ cups old-fashioned oats
- ✓ 1 ½ cups chopped walnuts
- ✓ ½ cup shelled sunflower seeds
- ✓ 1 cup golden raisins
- ✓ 1 cup shaved almonds
- ✓ 1 cup pure maple syrup
- ✓ ½ tsp ground cinnamon
- ✓ ¼ tsp ground allspice
- ✓ A pinch of salt

Directions:

Preheat oven to 325 F. In a baking dish, place the oats, walnuts, and sunflower seeds. Bake for 10 minutes.

Lower the heat from the oven to 300 F. Stir in the raisins, almonds, maple syrup, cinnamon, allspice, and salt. Bake for an additional 15 minutes. Allow cooling before serving

18) EXOTIC PECAN AND PUMPKIN SEED OAT JARS

Preparation Time: 10 minutes + chilling time		Servings: 5

Ingredients:

- ✓ 2 ½ cups old-fashioned rolled oats
- ✓ 5 tbsp pumpkin seeds
- ✓ 5 tbsp chopped pecans
- ✓ 5 cups unsweetened soy milk
- ✓ 2 ½ tsp agave syrup
- ✓ Salt to taste
- ✓ 1 tsp ground cardamom
- ✓ 1 tsp ground ginger

Directions:

- In a bowl, put oats, pumpkin seeds, pecans, soy milk, agave syrup, salt, cardamom, and ginger and toss to combine. Divide the mixture between mason jars. Seal the lids and transfer to the fridge to soak for 10-12 hours

19) SWEET APPLE MUFFINS

Preparation Time: 40 minutes		Servings: 4

Ingredients:

- ✓ For the muffins:
- ✓ 1 flax seed powder + 3 tbsp water
- ✓ 1 ½ cups whole-wheat flour
- ✓ ¾ cup pure date sugar
- ✓ 2 tsp baking powder
- ✓ ¼ tsp salt
- ✓ 1 tsp cinnamon powder
- ✓ 1/3 cup melted plant butter
- ✓ 1/3 cup flax milk
- ✓ 2 apples, chopped
- ✓ For topping:
- ✓ 1/3 cup whole-wheat flour
- ✓ ½ cup pure date sugar
- ✓ ½ cup cold plant butter, cubed
- ✓ 1 ½ tsp cinnamon powder

Directions:

Preheat oven to 400 F and grease 6 muffin cups with cooking spray. In a bowl, mix the flax seed powder with water and allow thickening for 5 minutes to make the vegan "flax egg."

In a bowl, mix flour, date sugar, baking powder, salt, and cinnamon powder. Whisk in the butter, vegan "flax egg," flax milk, and fold in the apples. Fill the muffin cups two-thirds way up with the batter.

In a bowl, mix remaining flour, date sugar, cold butter, and cinnamon powder. Sprinkle the mixture on the muffin batter. Bake for 20 minutes. Remove the muffins onto a wire rack, allow cooling, and serve

20) ALMOND GREEK YOGURT WITH BERRIES AND WALNUTS

Preparation Time: 10 minutes		Servings: 4

Ingredients:

- ✓ 4 cups almond milk
- ✓ Dairy-Free yogurt, cold
- ✓ 2 tbsp pure malt syrup
- ✓ 2 cups mixed berries, chopped
- ✓ ¼ cup chopped toasted walnuts

Directions:

In a medium bowl, mix the yogurt and malt syrup until well-combined. Divide the mixture into 4 breakfast bowls. Top with the berries and walnuts. Enjoy immediately

21) SPECIAL BREAKFAST BLUEBERRY MUESLI

Preparation Time: 10 minutes		Servings: 5

Ingredients:

- ✓ 2 cups spelt flakes
- ✓ 2 cups puffed cereal
- ✓ ¼ cup sunflower seeds
- ✓ ¼ cup almonds
- ✓ ¼ cup raisins
- ✓ ¼ cup dried cranberries
- ✓ ¼ cup chopped dried figs
- ✓ ¼ cup shredded coconut
- ✓ ¼ cup non-dairy chocolate chips
- ✓ 3 tsp ground cinnamon
- ✓ ½ cup coconut milk
- ✓ ½ cup blueberries

Directions:

- In a bowl, combine the spelt flakes, puffed cereal, sunflower seeds, almonds, raisins, cranberries, figs, coconut, chocolate chips, and cinnamon. Toss to mix well. Pour in the coconut milk. Let sit for 1 hour and serve topped with blueberries

22) QUICK BERRY AND ALMOND BUTTER SWIRL BOWL

Preparation Time: 10 minutes		Servings: 3

Ingredients:

- ✓ 1 ½ cups almond milk
- ✓ 2 small bananas
- ✓ 2 cups mixed berries, fresh or frozen
- ✓ 3 dates, pitted
- ✓ 3 scoops hemp protein powder
- ✓ 3 tbsp smooth almond butter
- ✓ 2 tbsp pepitas

Directions:

In your blender or food processor, mix the almond milk with the bananas, berries and dates.

Process until everything is well combined. Divide the smoothie between three bowls.

Top each smoothie bowl with almond butter and use a butter knife to swirl the almond butter into the top of each smoothie bowl.

Afterwards, garnish each smoothie bowl with pepitas, serve well-chilled and enjoy

23) EXOTIC OATS WITH COCONUT AND STRAWBERRIES

Preparation Time: 15 minutes		Servings: 2

Ingredients:

- ✓ 1/2 tbsp coconut oil
- ✓ 1 cup rolled oats
- ✓ A pinch of flaky sea salt
- ✓ 1/8 tsp grated nutmeg
- ✓ 1/4 tsp cardamom
- ✓ 1 tbsp coconut sugar
- ✓ 1 cup coconut milk, sweetened
- ✓ 1 cup water
- ✓ 2 tbsp coconut flakes
- ✓ 4 tbsp fresh strawberries

Directions:

In a saucepan, melt the coconut oil over a moderate flame. Then, toast the oats for about 3 minutes, stirring continuously.

Add in the salt, nutmeg, cardamom, coconut sugar, milk and water; continue to cook for 12 minutes more or until cooked through.

Spoon the mixture into serving bowls; top with coconut flakes and fresh strawberries. Enjoy

24) BEST ITALIAN CHOCOLATE GRANOLA

Preparation Time: 1 hour | | **Servings:** 10

Ingredients:

- ✓ 1/2 cup coconut oil
- ✓ 1/2 cup agave syrup
- ✓ 1 tsp vanilla paste
- ✓ 3 cups rolled oats
- ✓ 1/2 cup hazelnuts, chopped
- ✓ 1/2 cup pumpkin seeds

- ✓ 1/2 tsp ground cardamom
- ✓ 1 tsp ground cinnamon
- ✓ 1/4 tsp ground cloves
- ✓ 1 tsp Himalayan salt
- ✓ 1/2 cup dark chocolate, cut into chunks

Directions:

Begin by preheating your oven to 260 degrees F; line two rimmed baking sheets with a piece parchment paper.

Then, thoroughly combine the coconut oil, agave syrup and vanilla in a mixing bowl.

Gradually add in the oats, hazelnuts, pumpkin seeds and spices; toss to coat well. Spread the mixture out onto the prepared baking sheets.

Bake in the middle of the oven, stirring halfway through the cooking time, for about 1 hour or until golden brown.

Stir in the dark chocolate and let your granola cool completely before storing. Store in an airtight container.

Enjoy

25) ENGLISH PUMPKIN GRIDDLE CAKES AUTUMN SEASON

Preparation Time: 30 minutes | | **Servings:** 4

Ingredients:

- ✓ 1/2 cup oat flour
- ✓ 1/2 cup whole-wheat white flour
- ✓ 1 tsp baking powder
- ✓ 1/4 tsp Himalayan salt
- ✓ 1 tsp sugar
- ✓ 1/2 tsp ground allspice

- ✓ 1/2 tsp ground cinnamon
- ✓ 1/2 tsp crystalized ginger
- ✓ 1 tsp lemon juice, freshly squeezed
- ✓ 1/2 cup almond milk
- ✓ 1/2 cup pumpkin puree
- ✓ 2 tbsp coconut oil

Directions:

In a mixing bowl, thoroughly combine the flour, baking powder, salt, sugar and spices. Gradually add in the lemon juice, milk and pumpkin puree.

Heat an electric griddle on medium and lightly slick it with the coconut oil.

Cook your cake for approximately 3 minutes until the bubbles form; flip it and cook on the other side for 3 minutes longer until browned on the underside.

Repeat with the remaining oil and batter. Serve dusted with cinnamon sugar, if desired. Enjoy

26) GREEK MUFFINS WITH TOFU ENGLISH RECIPE

Preparation Time: 15 minutes | | **Servings:** 4

Ingredients:

- ✓ 2 tbsp olive oil
- ✓ 16 ounces extra-firm tofu
- ✓ 1 tbsp nutritional yeast
- ✓ 1/4 tsp turmeric powder
- ✓ 2 handfuls fresh kale, chopped

- ✓ Kosher salt and ground black pepper, to taste
- ✓ 4 English muffins, cut in half
- ✓ 4 tbsp ketchup
- ✓ 4 slices vegan cheese

Directions:

Heat the olive oil in a frying skillet over medium heat. When it's hot, add the tofu and sauté for 8 minutes, stirring occasionally to promote even cooking.

Add in the nutritional yeast, turmeric and kale and continue sautéing an additional 2 minutes or until the kale wilts. Season with salt and pepper to taste.

Meanwhile, toast the English muffins until crisp.

To assemble the sandwiches, spread the bottom halves of the English muffins with ketchup; top them with the tofu mixture and vegan cheese; place the bun topper on, close the sandwiches and serve warm.

Enjoy

27) SPECIAL CINNAMON SEMOLINO PORRIDGE

Preparation Time: 20 minutes		Servings: 3

Ingredients:	✓ 1/4 tsp kosher salt ✓ 1/2 tsp ground cinnamon ✓ 1 ¼ cups semolina	Directions:
✓ 3 cups almond milk ✓ 3 tbsp maple syrup ✓ 3 tsp coconut oil		In a saucepan, heat the almond milk, maple syrup, coconut oil, salt and cinnamon over a moderate flame. Once hot, gradually stir in the semolina flour. Turn the heat to a simmer and continue cooking until the porridge reaches your preferred consistency. Garnish with your favorite toppings and serve warm. Enjoy

28) EASY APPLESAUCE DECADENT FRENCH TOAST

Preparation Time: 15 minutes		Servings: 1

Ingredients:	✓ 1/4 tsp ground cloves ✓ 1/4 tsp ground cinnamon ✓ 2 slices rustic day-old bread slices ✓ 1 tbsp coconut oil ✓ 1 tbsp maple syrup	Directions:
✓ 1/4 cup oat milk, sweetened ✓ 2 tbsp applesauce, sweetened ✓ 1/2 tsp vanilla paste ✓ A pinch of salt ✓ A pinch of grated nutmeg		In a mixing bowl, thoroughly combine the oat milk, applesauce, vanilla, salt, nutmeg, cloves and cinnamon. Dip each slice of bread into the custard mixture until well coated on all sides. Preheat the coconut oil in a frying pan over medium-high heat. Cook for about 3 minutes on each side, until golden brown. Drizzle the French toast with maple syrup and serve immediately. Enjoy

29) TASTY NUTTY BREAKFAST BREAD PUDDING

Preparation Time: 2 hours 10 minutes		Servings: 6

Ingredients:	✓ 1/2 tsp ground cinnamon ✓ 1/2 tsp ground cloves ✓ 1/3 tsp kosher salt ✓ 1/2 cup almonds, roughly chopped ✓ 4 cups day-old white bread, cubed	Directions:
✓ 1 ½ cups almond milk ✓ 1/2 cup maple syrup ✓ 2 tbsp almond butter ✓ 1/2 tsp vanilla extract ✓ 1/2 tsp almond extract		In a mixing bowl, combine the almond milk, maple syrup, almond butter, vanilla extract, almond extract and spices. Add the bread cubes to the custard mixture and stir to combine well. Fold in the almonds and allow it to rest for about 1 hour. Then, spoon the mixture into a lightly oiled casserole dish. Bake in the preheated oven at 350 degrees F for about 1 hour or until the top is golden brown. Place the bread pudding on a wire rack for 10 minutes before slicing and serving. Enjoy

30) FRITTATA WITH MUSHROOMS AND PEPPERS

Preparation Time: 30 minutes | | **Servings:** 4

Ingredients:

- ✓ 4 tbsp olive oil
- ✓ 1 red onion, minced
- ✓ 1 red bell pepper, sliced
- ✓ 1 tsp garlic, finely chopped
- ✓ 1 pound button mushrooms, sliced
- ✓ Sea salt and ground black pepper, to taste
- ✓ 1/2 tsp dried oregano
- ✓ 1/2 tsp dried dill
- ✓ 16 ounces tofu, drained and crumbled
- ✓ 2 tbsp nutritional yeast
- ✓ 1/2 tsp turmeric powder
- ✓ 4 tbsp corn flour
- ✓ 1/3 cup oat milk, unsweetened

Directions:

- ❖ Preheat 2 tbsp of the olive oil in a nonstick skillet over medium-high heat. Then, cook the onion and pepper for about 4 minutes until tender and fragrant.
- ❖ Add in the garlic and mushrooms and continue to sauté an additional 2 to 3 minutes or until aromatic. Season with salt, black pepper, oregano and dill. Reserve.
- ❖ In your blender or food processor, mix the tofu, nutritional yeast, turmeric powder, corn flour and milk. Process until you have a smooth and uniform paste.
- ❖ In the same skillet, heat 1 tbsp of the olive oil until sizzling. Pour in 1/2 of the tofu mixture and spread it with a spatula.
- ❖ Cook for about 6 minutes or until set; flip and cook it for another 3 minutes. Slide the omelet onto a serving plate.
- ❖ Spoon 1/2 of the mushroom filling over half of the omelet. Fold the unfilled half of omelet over the filling.
- ❖ Repeat with another omelet. Cut them into halves and serve warm. Enjoy

31) FROZEN HEMP AND BLACKBERRY SMOOTHIE BOWL

Preparation Time: 10 minutes | | **Servings:** 2

Ingredients:

- ✓ 2 tbsp hemp seeds
- ✓ 1/2 cup coconut milk
- ✓ 1 cup coconut yogurt
- ✓ 1 cup blackberries, frozen
- ✓ 2 small-sized bananas, frozen
- ✓ 4 tbsp granola

Directions:

- ❖ In your blender, mix all ingredients, trying to keep the liquids at the bottom of the blender to help it break up the fruits.
- ❖ Divide your smoothie between serving bowls.
- ❖ Garnish each bowl with granola and some extra frozen berries, if desired. Serve immediately

32) DARK CHOCOLATE AND WALNUT STEEL-CUT OATS

Preparation Time: 30 minutes | | **Servings:** 3

Ingredients:

- ✓ 2 cups oat milk
- ✓ 1/3 cup steel-cut oats
- ✓ 1 tbsp coconut oil
- ✓ 1/4 cup coconut sugar
- ✓ A pinch of grated nutmeg
- ✓ A pinch of flaky sea salt
- ✓ 1/4 tsp cinnamon powder
- ✓ 1/4 tsp vanilla extract
- ✓ 4 tbsp cocoa powder
- ✓ 1/3 cup English walnut halves
- ✓ 4 tbsp chocolate chips

Directions:

- ❖ Bring the oat milk and oats to a boil over a moderately high heat. Then, turn the heat to low and add in the coconut oil, sugar and spices; let it simmer for about 25 minutes, stirring periodically.
- ❖ Add in the cocoa powder and continue simmering an additional 3 minutes.
- ❖ Spoon the oatmeal into serving bowls. Top each bowl with the walnut halves and chocolate chips.
- ❖ Enjoy
- ❖

33) EASY BUCKWHEAT PORRIDGE WITH APPLES-ALMONDS

Preparation Time: 20 minutes		Servings: 3

Ingredients:

- ✓ 1 cup buckwheat groats, toasted
- ✓ 3/4 cup water
- ✓ 1 cup rice milk
- ✓ 1/4 tsp sea salt
- ✓ 3 tbsp agave syrup
- ✓ 1 cup apples, cored and diced
- ✓ 3 tbsp almonds, slivered
- ✓ 2 tbsp coconut flakes
- ✓ 2 tbsp hemp seeds

Directions:

- ❖ In a saucepan, bring the buckwheat groats, water, milk and salt to a boil. Immediately turn the heat to a simmer; let it simmer for about 13 minutes until it has softened.
- ❖ Stir in the agave syrup. Divide the porridge between three serving bowls.
- ❖ Garnish each serving with the apples, almonds, coconut and hemp seeds. Enjoy

34) TRADITIONAL SPANISH TORTILLA

Preparation Time: 35 minutes		Servings: 2

Ingredients:

- ✓ 3 tbsp olive oil
- ✓ 2 medium potatoes, peeled and diced
- ✓ 1/2 white onion, chopped
- ✓ 8 tbsp gram flour
- ✓ 8 tbsp water
- ✓ Sea salt and ground black pepper, to season
- ✓ 1/2 tsp Spanish paprika

Directions:

- ❖ Heat 2 tbsp of the olive oil in a frying pan over a moderate flame. Now, cook the potatoes and onion; cook for about 20 minutes or until tender; reserve.
- ❖ In a mixing bowl, thoroughly combine the flour, water, salt, black pepper and paprika. Add in the potato/onion mixture.
- ❖ Heat the remaining 1 tbsp of the olive oil in the same frying pan. Pour 1/2 of the batter into the frying pan. Cook your tortilla for about 11 minutes, turning it once or twice to promote even cooking.
- ❖ Repeat with the remaining batter and serve warm

35) SPECIAL CHOCOLATE AND MANGO QUINOA BOWL

Preparation Time: 35 minutes		Servings: 2

Ingredients:

- ✓ 1 cup quinoa
- ✓ 1 tsp ground cinnamon
- ✓ 1 cup non-dairy milk
- ✓ 1 large mango, chopped
- ✓ 3 tbsp unsweetened cocoa powder
- ✓ 2 tbsp almond butter
- ✓ 1 tbsp hemp seeds
- ✓ 1 tbsp walnuts
- ✓ ¼ cup raspberries

Directions:

- ❖ In a pot, combine the quinoa, cinnamon, milk, and 1 cup of water over medium heat. Bring to a boil, low heat, and simmer covered for 25-30 minutes. In a bowl, mash the mango and mix cocoa powder, almond butter, and hemp seeds. In a serving bowl, place cooked quinoa and mango mixture.
- ❖ Top with walnuts and raspberries. Serve immediately

36) EASY ORANGE AND CARROT MUFFINS WITH CHERRIES

Preparation Time: 45 minutes		Servings: 6

- ✓ 1 tsp vegetable oil
- ✓ 2 tbsp almond butter
- ✓ ¼ cup non-dairy milk
- ✓ 1 orange, peeled
- ✓ 1 carrot, coarsely chopped
- ✓ 2 tbsp chopped dried cherries
- ✓ 3 tbsp molasses
- ✓ 2 tbsp ground flaxseed
- ✓ 1 tsp apple cider vinegar
- ✓ 1 tsp pure vanilla extract
- ✓ ½ tsp ground cinnamon
- ✓ ½ tsp ground ginger
- ✓ ¼ tsp ground nutmeg
- ✓ ¼ tsp allspice
- ✓ ¾ cup whole-wheat flour
- ✓ 1 tsp baking powder
- ✓ ½ tsp baking soda
- ✓ ½ cup rolled oats
- ✓ 2 tbsp raisins
- ✓ 2 tbsp sunflower seeds

Directions:

- ❖ Preheat oven to 350 F. Grease 6 muffin cups with vegetable oil.
- ❖ In a food processor, add the almond butter, milk, orange, carrot, cherries, molasses, flaxseed, vinegar, vanilla, cinnamon, ginger, nutmeg, and allspice and blend until smooth.
- ❖ In a bowl, combine the flour, baking powder, and baking soda. Fold in the wet mixture and gently stir to combine. Mix in the oats, raisins, and sunflower seeds. Divide the batter between muffin cups. Put in a baking tray and bake for 30 minutes

37) SIMPLE QUINOA LEMONY MUFFINS

Preparation Time: 25 minutes		Servings: 5

Ingredients:

- ✓ 2 tbsp coconut oil melted, plus more for coating the muffin tin
- ✓ ¼ cup ground flaxseed
- ✓ 2 cups unsweetened lemon curd
- ✓ ½ cup pure date sugar
- ✓ 1 tsp apple cider vinegar
- ✓ 2 ½ cups whole-wheat flour
- ✓ 1 ½ cups cooked quinoa
- ✓ 2 tsp baking soda
- ✓ A pinch of salt
- ✓ ½ cup raisins

Directions:

- ❖ Preheat oven to 400 F.
- ❖ In a bowl, combine the flaxseed and ½ cup water. Stir in the lemon curd, sugar, coconut oil, and vinegar. Add in flour, quinoa, baking soda, and salt. Put in the raisins, be careful not too fluffy.
- ❖ Divide the batter between greased with coconut oil cups of the tin and bake for 20 minutes until golden and set. Allow cooling slightly before removing it from the tin. Serve

38) RICH OATMEAL ALMOND PORRIDGE

Preparation Time: 25 minutes		Servings: 4

Ingredients:

- ✓ 2 ½ cups vegetable broth
- ✓ 2 ½ cups almond milk
- ✓ ½ cup steel-cut oats
- ✓ 1 tbsp pearl barley
- ✓ ½ cup slivered almonds
- ✓ ¼ cup nutritional yeast
- ✓ 2 cups old-fashioned rolled oats

Directions:

- ❖ • Pour the broth and almond milk in a pot over medium heat and bring to a boil. Stir in oats, pearl barley, almond slivers, and nutritional yeast. Reduce the heat and simmer for 20 minutes. Add in the rolled oats, cook for an additional 5 minutes, until creamy. Allow cooling before serving

39) RICH BREAKFAST PECAN AND PEAR FARRO

Preparation Time: 20 minutes		Servings: 4

Ingredients:

- ✓ 2 cups water
- ✓ ½ tsp salt
- ✓ 1 cup farro
- ✓ 1 tbsp plant butter
- ✓ 2 pears, peeled, cored, and chopped
- ✓ ¼ cup chopped pecans

Directions:

- ❖ Bring water to a boil in a pot over high heat. Stir in salt and farro. Lower the heat, cover, and simmer for 15 minutes until the farro is tender and the liquid has absorbed. Turn the heat off and add in the butter, pears, and pecans. Cover and rest for 12-15 minutes.
- ❖ Serve immediately

40) SIMPLE BLACKBERRY WAFFLES

Preparation Time: 15 minutes		Servings: 4

Ingredients:

- ✓ 1 ½ cups whole-heat flour
- ✓ ½ cup old-fashioned oats
- ✓ ¼ cup date sugar
- ✓ 3 tsp baking powder
- ✓ ½ tsp salt
- ✓ 1 tsp ground cinnamon
- ✓ 2 cups soy milk
- ✓ 1 tbsp fresh lemon juice
- ✓ 1 tsp lemon zest
- ✓ ¼ cup plant butter, melted
- ✓ ½ cup fresh blackberries

Directions:

- ❖ Preheat the waffle iron.
- ❖ In a bowl, mix flour, oats, sugar, baking powder, salt, and cinnamon. Set aside. In another bowl, combine milk, lemon juice, lemon zest, and butter. Pour into the wet ingredients and whisk to combine. Add the batter to the hot greased waffle iron, using approximately a ladleful for each waffle. Cook for 3-5 minutes, until golden brown. Repeat the process until no batter is left.
- ❖ Serve topped with blackberries

41) AUTHENTIC WALNUT WAFFLES WITH MAPLE SYRUP

Preparation Time: 15 minutes		Servings: 4

Ingredients:

- ✓ 1 ¾ cups whole-wheat flour
- ✓ ⅓ cup coarsely ground walnuts
- ✓ 1 tbsp baking powder
- ✓ 1 ½p cups soy milk
- ✓ 3 tbsp pure maple syrup
- ✓ 3 tbsp plant butter, melted

Directions:

- ❖ Preheat the waffle iron and grease with oil. Combine the flour, walnuts, baking powder, and salt in a bowl. Set aside. In another bowl, mix the milk and butter. Pour into the walnut mixture and whisk until well combined. Spoon a ladleful of the batter onto the waffle iron.
- ❖ Cook for 3-5 minutes, until golden brown. Repeat the process until no batter is left. Top with maple syrup to serve

42) SIMPLE ORANGE AND BRAN CUPS WITH DATES

Preparation Time: 30 minutes		Servings: 12

Ingredients:

- ✓ 1 tsp vegetable oil
- ✓ 3 cups bran flakes cereal
- ✓ 1 ½ cups whole-wheat flour
- ✓ ½ cup dates, chopped
- ✓ 3 tsp baking powder
- ✓ ½ tsp ground cinnamon
- ✓ ½ tsp salt
- ✓ ⅓ cup brown sugar
- ✓ ¾ cup fresh orange juice

Directions:

- ❖ Preheat oven to 400 F. Grease a 12-cup muffin tin with oil.
- ❖ Mix the bran flakes, flour, dates, baking powder, cinnamon, and salt in a bowl. In another bowl, combine the sugar and orange juice until blended. Pour into the dry mixture and whisk. Divide the mixture between the cups of the muffin tin. Bake for 20 minutes or until golden brown and set. Cool for a few minutes before removing from the tin and serve

43) EXOTIC MACADAMIA NUTS AND APPLE-DATE COUSCOUS

Preparation Time: 20 minutes		Servings: 4

Ingredients:

- ✓ 3 cups apple juice
- ✓ 1 ½ cups couscous
- ✓ 1 tsp ground cinnamon
- ✓ ¼ tsp ground cloves
- ✓ ½ cup dried dates
- ✓ ½ cup chopped macadamia nuts

Directions:

- ❖ Pour the apple juice into a pot over medium heat and bring to a boil. Stir in couscous, cinnamon, and cloves. Turn the heat off and cover. Let sit for 5 minutes until the liquid is absorbed.
- ❖ Using a fork, fluff the couscous and add the dates and macadamia nuts, stir to combine. Serve warm

44) TASTY BLUEBERRY COCONUT MUFFINS

Preparation Time: 30 minutes		Servings: 12

Ingredients:

- ✓ 1 tbsp coconut oil melted
- ✓ 1 cup quick-cooking oats
- ✓ 1 cup boiling water
- ✓ ½ cup almond milk
- ✓ ¼ cup ground flaxseed
- ✓ 1 tsp almond extract
- ✓ 1 tsp apple cider vinegar
- ✓ 1 ½ cups whole-wheat flour
- ✓ ½ cup pure date sugar
- ✓ 2 tsp baking soda
- ✓ A pinch of salt
- ✓ 1 cup blueberries

Directions:

- ❖ Preheat oven to 400 F.
- ❖ In a bowl, stir in the oats with boiling water until they are softened. Pour in the coconut oil, milk, flaxseed, almond extract, and vinegar. Add in the flour, sugar, baking soda, and salt. Gently stir in blueberries.
- ❖ Divide the batter between a greased with coconut oil muffin tin. Bake for 20 minutes until lightly brown. Allow cooling for 10 minutes. Using a spatula, run the sides of the muffins to take out. Serve

45) SWISS-STYLE CHARD SCRAMBLED TOFU

Preparation Time: 35 minutes		Servings: 5

Ingredients:

- ✓ 1 (14-oz) package tofu, crumbled
- ✓ 2 tsp olive oil
- ✓ 1 onion, chopped
- ✓ 3 cloves minced garlic
- ✓ 1 celery stalk, chopped
- ✓ 2 large carrots, chopped
- ✓ 1 tsp chili powder
- ✓ ½ tsp ground cumin
- ✓ ½ tsp ground turmeric
- ✓ Salt and black pepper to taste
- ✓ 5 cups Swiss chard

Directions:

- ❖ Heat the oil in a skillet over medium heat. Add in the onion, garlic, celery, and carrots. Sauté for 5 minutes. Stir in tofu, chili powder, cumin, turmeric, salt, and pepper, cook for 7-8 minutes more.
- ❖ Mix in the Swiss chard and cook until wilted, about 3 minutes. Allow cooling and seal and serve

46) BEST BAKED SPICY EGGPLANT

Preparation Time: 30 minutes		Servings: 4

Ingredients:

- ✓ 2 large eggplants
- ✓ Salt and black pepper to taste
- ✓ 2 tbsp plant butter
- ✓ 1 tsp red chili flakes
- ✓ 4 oz raw ground almonds

Directions:

- ❖ Preheat oven to 400 F.
- ❖ Cut off the head of the eggplants and slice the body into 2-inch rounds. Season with salt and black pepper and arrange on a parchment paper-lined baking sheet.
- ❖ Drop thin slices of the plant butter on each eggplant slice, sprinkle with red chili flakes, and bake in the oven for 20 minutes.
- ❖ Slide the baking sheet out and sprinkle with the almonds. Roast further for 5 minutes or until golden brown. Dish the eggplants and serve with arugula salad

47) VERY GOOD MASHED BROCCOLI WITH ROASTED GARLIC

Preparation Time: 45 minutes		Servings: 4

Ingredients:

- ✓ ½ head garlic
- ✓ 2 tbsp olive oil + for garnish
- ✓ 1 head broccoli, cut into florets
- ✓ 1 tsp salt
- ✓ 4 oz plant butter
- ✓ ¼ tsp dried thyme
- ✓ Juice and zest of half a lemon
- ✓ 4 tbsp coconut cream

Directions:

- ❖ Preheat oven to 400 F.
- ❖ Use a knife to cut a ¼ inch off the top of the garlic cloves, drizzle with olive oil, and wrap in aluminum foil. Place on a baking sheet and roast for 30 minutes. Remove and set aside when ready.
- ❖ Pour the broccoli into a pot, add 3 cups of water, and 1 tsp of salt. Bring to a boil until tender, about 7 minutes. Drain and transfer the broccoli to a bowl. Add the plant butter, thyme, lemon juice and zest, coconut cream, and olive oil. Use an immersion blender to puree the ingredients until smooth and nice. Spoon the mash into serving bowls and garnish with some olive oil. Serve

48) SIMPLE SPICY PISTACHIO DIP

Preparation Time: 10 minutes		Servings: 4

Ingredients:

- ✓ 3 oz toasted pistachios + for garnish
- ✓ 3 tbsp coconut cream
- ✓ ¼ cup water
- ✓ Juice of half a lemon
- ✓ ½ tsp smoked paprika
- ✓ Cayenne pepper to taste
- ✓ ½ tsp salt
- ✓ ½ cup olive oil

Directions:

- ❖ Pour the pistachios, coconut cream, water, lemon juice, paprika, cayenne pepper, and salt. Puree the ingredients at high speed until smooth. Add the olive oil and puree a little further. Manage the consistency of the dip by adding more oil or water. Spoon the dip into little bowls, garnish with some pistachios, and serve with julienned celery and carrots

49) HUNGARIAN PAPRIKA ROASTED NUTS

Preparation Time: 10 minutes		Servings: 4
✓ 8 oz walnuts and pecans ✓ 1 tsp salt ✓ 1 tbsp coconut oil	✓ 1 tsp cumin powder ✓ 1 tsp paprika powder	❖ In a bowl, mix walnuts, pecans, salt, coconut oil, cumin powder, and paprika powder until the nuts are well coated with spice and oil. Pour the mixture into a pan and toast while stirring continually. Once the nuts are fragrant and brown, transfer to a bowl. Allow cooling and serve with a chilled berry juice

50) EASY MIXED VEGETABLES WITH BASIL

Preparation Time: 40 minutes		Servings: 4
Ingredients: ✓ 2 medium zucchinis, chopped ✓ 2 medium yellow squash, chopped ✓ 1 red onion, cut into 1-inch wedges ✓ 1 red bell pepper, diced ✓ 1 cup cherry tomatoes, halved	✓ 4 tbsp olive oil ✓ Salt and black pepper to taste ✓ 3 garlic cloves, minced ✓ 2/3 cup whole-wheat breadcrumbs ✓ 1 lemon, zested ✓ ¼ cup chopped fresh basil	❖ Preheat the oven to 450 F. Lightly grease a large baking sheet with cooking spray. ❖ In a medium bowl, add the zucchini, yellow squash, red onion, bell pepper, tomatoes, olive oil, salt, black pepper, and garlic. Toss well and spread the mixture on the baking sheet. Roast in the oven for 25 to 30 minutes or until the vegetables are tender while stirring every 5 minutes. ❖ Meanwhile, heat the olive oil in a medium skillet and sauté the garlic until fragrant. Mix in the breadcrumbs, lemon zest, and basil. Cook for 2 to 3 minutes. Remove the vegetables from the oven and toss in the breadcrumb's mixture. Serve

51) DELICIOUS ONION RINGS AND KALE DIP

Preparation Time: 35 minutes		Servings: 4
Ingredients: ✓ 1 onion, sliced into rings ✓ 1 tbsp flaxseed meal + 3 tbsp water ✓ 1 cup almond flour ✓ ½ cup grated plant-based Parmesan ✓ 2 tsp garlic powder ✓ ½ tbsp sweet paprika powder	✓ 2 oz chopped kale ✓ 2 tbsp olive oil ✓ 2 tbsp dried cilantro ✓ 1 tbsp dried oregano ✓ Salt and black pepper to taste ✓ 1 cup tofu mayonnaise ✓ 4 tbsp coconut cream ✓ Juice of ½ a lemon	❖ Preheat oven to 400 F. In a bowl, mix the flaxseed meal and water and leave the mixture to thicken and fully absorb for 5 minutes. In another bowl, combine almond flour, plant-based Parmesan cheese, half of the garlic powder, sweet paprika, and salt. Line a baking sheet with parchment paper in readiness for the rings. When the vegan "flax egg" is ready, dip in the onion rings one after another, and then into the almond flour mixture. Place the rings on the baking sheet and grease with cooking spray. Bake for 15-20 minutes or until golden brown and crispy. Remove the onion rings into a serving bowl. Put kale in a food processor. Add in olive oil, cilantro, oregano, remaining garlic powder, salt, black pepper, tofu mayonnaise, coconut cream, and lemon juice; puree until nice and smooth. Allow the dip to sit for about 10 minutes for the flavors to develop. After, serve the dip with the crispy onion rings

52) PORTUGUESE SOY CHORIZO STUFFED CABBAGE ROLLS

Preparation Time: 35 minutes		Servings: 4
Ingredients: ✓ ¼ cup coconut oil, divided ✓ 1 large white onion, chopped ✓ 3 cloves garlic, minced, divided ✓ 1 cup crumbled soy chorizo	✓ 1 cup cauliflower rice ✓ 1 can tomato sauce ✓ 1 tsp dried oregano ✓ 1 tsp dried basil ✓ 8 full green cabbage leaves	❖ Heat half of the coconut oil in a saucepan over medium heat. ❖ Add half of the onion, half of the garlic, and all of the soy chorizo. Sauté for 5 minutes or until the chorizo has browned further, and the onion softened. Stir in the cauli rice, season with salt and black pepper, and cook for 3 to 4 minutes. Turn the heat off and set the pot aside. Heat the remaining oil in a saucepan over medium heat, add, and sauté the remaining onion and garlic until fragrant and soft. Pour in the tomato sauce, and season with salt, black pepper, oregano, and basil. Add ¼ cup water and simmer the sauce for 10 minutes. While the sauce cooks, lay the cabbage leaves on a flat surface and spoon the soy chorizo mixture into the middle of each leaf. Roll the leaves to secure the filling. Place the cabbage rolls in the tomato sauce and cook further for 10 minutes. When ready, serve the cabbage rolls with sauce over mashed broccoli or with mixed seed bread

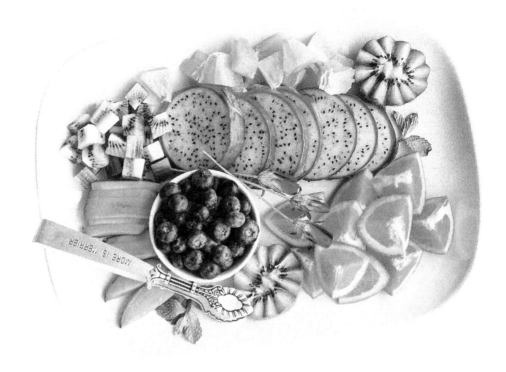

53) TROPICAL BANANA TANGERINE TOAST

Preparation Time: 25 minutes		Servings: 4

Ingredients:

- ✓ 3 bananas
- ✓ 1 cup almond milk
- ✓ Zest and juice of 1 tangerine
- ✓ 1 tsp ground cinnamon
- ✓ ¼ tsp grated nutmeg
- ✓ 4 slices bread
- ✓ 1 tbsp olive oil

Directions:

❖ Blend the bananas, almond milk, tangerine juice, tangerine zest, cinnamon, and nutmeg until smooth in a food processor. Spread into a baking dish. Submerge the bread slices in the mixture for 3-4 minutes.

❖ Heat the oil in a skillet over medium heat. Fry the bread for 5 minutes until golden brown. Serve hot

54) EASY MAPLE BANANA OATS

Preparation Time: 35 minutes		Servings: 4

Ingredients:

- ✓ 3 cups water
- ✓ 1 cup steel-cut oats
- ✓ 2 bananas, mashed
- ✓ ¼ cup pumpkin seeds
- ✓ 2 tbsp maple syrup
- ✓ A pinch of salt

Directions:

❖ Bring water to a boil in a pot, add in oats, and lower the heat. Cook for 20-30 minutes. Put in the mashed bananas, cook for 3-5 minutes more. Stir in maple syrup, pumpkin seeds, and salt. Serve

55) TASTY GINGERBREAD BELGIAN WAFFLES

Preparation Time: 25 minutes		Servings: 3

Ingredients:

- ✓ 1 cup all-purpose flour
- ✓ 1 tsp baking powder
- ✓ 1 tbsp brown sugar
- ✓ 1 tsp ground ginger
- ✓ 1 cup almond milk
- ✓ 1 tsp vanilla extract
- ✓ 2 olive oil

Directions:

- ❖ Preheat a waffle iron according to the manufacturer's instructions.
- ❖ In a mixing bowl, thoroughly combine the flour, baking powder, brown sugar, ground ginger, almond milk, vanilla extract and olive oil.
- ❖ Beat until everything is well blended.
- ❖ Ladle 1/3 of the batter into the preheated waffle iron and cook until the waffles are golden and crisp. Repeat with the remaining batter.
- ❖ Serve your waffles with blackberry jam, if desired. Enjoy

56) EASY BANANA AND WALNUTS PORRIDGE

Preparation Time: 15 minutes		Servings: 4

Ingredients:

- ✓ 1 cup rolled oats
- ✓ 1 cup spelt flakes
- ✓ 2 cups unsweetened almond milk
- ✓ 4 tbsp agave nectar
- ✓ 4 tbsp walnuts, chopped
- ✓ 2 bananas, sliced

Directions:

- ❖ In a nonstick skillet, fry the oats and spelt flakes until fragrant, working in batches.
- ❖ Bring the milk to a boil and add in the oats, spelt flakes and agave nectar.
- ❖ Turn the heat to a simmer and let it cook for 6 to 7 minutes, stirring occasionally. Top with walnuts and bananas and serve warm. Enjoy

Chapter 2.

LUNCH

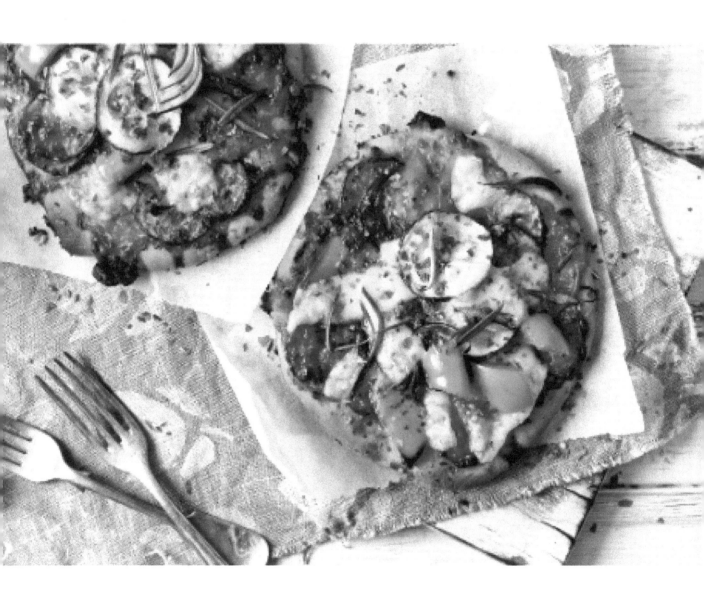

57) DELICIOUS GARLIC CROSTINI WITH CABBAGE SOUP

Preparation Time: 1 hour		Servings: 4

Ingredients:

- Soup:
- 2 tbsp olive oil
- 1 medium leek, chopped
- 1 cup turnip, chopped
- 1 parsnip, chopped
- 1 carrot, chopped
- 2 cups cabbage, shredded
- 2 garlic cloves, finely chopped
- 4 cups vegetable broth
- 2 bay leaves
- Sea salt and ground black pepper, to taste
- 1/4 tsp cumin seeds
- 1/2 tsp mustard seeds
- 1 tsp dried basil
- 2 tomatoes, pureed
- Crostini:
- 8 slices of baguette
- 2 heads garlic
- 4 tbsp extra-virgin olive oil

Directions:

In a soup pot, heat 2 tbsp of the olive over medium-high heat. Now, sauté the leek, turnip, parsnip and carrot for about 4 minutes or until the vegetables are crisp-tender.

Add in the garlic and cabbage and continue to sauté for 1 minute or until aromatic.

Then, stir in the vegetable broth, bay leaves, salt, black pepper, cumin seeds, mustard seeds, dried basil and pureed tomatoes; bring to a boil. Immediately reduce the heat to a simmer and let it cook for about 20 minutes.

Meanwhile, preheat your oven to 375 degrees F. Now, roast the garlic and baguette slices for about 15 minutes. Remove the crostini from the oven.

Continue baking the garlic for 45 minutes more or until very tender. Allow the garlic to cool.

Now, cut each head of the garlic using a sharp serrated knife in order to separate all the cloves.

Squeeze the roasted garlic cloves out of their skins. Mash the garlic pulp with 4 tbsp of the extra-virgin olive oil.

Spread the roasted garlic mixture evenly on the tops of the crostini. Serve with the warm soup. Enjoy

58) TASTY GREEN BEAN SOUP CREAM

Preparation Time: 35 minutes		Servings: 4

Ingredients:

- 1 tbsp sesame oil
- 1 onion, chopped
- 1 green pepper, seeded and chopped
- 2 russet potatoes, peeled and diced
- 2 garlic cloves, chopped
- 4 cups vegetable broth
- 1 pound green beans, trimmed
- Sea salt and ground black pepper, to season
- 1 cup full-fat coconut milk

Directions:

In a heavy-bottomed pot, heat the sesame over medium-high heat. Now, sauté the onion, peppers and potatoes for about 5 minutes, stirring periodically.

Add in the garlic and continue sautéing for 1 minute or until fragrant.

Then, stir in the vegetable broth, green beans, salt and black pepper; bring to a boil. Immediately reduce the heat to a simmer and let it cook for 20 minutes.

Puree the green bean mixture using an immersion blender until creamy and uniform.

Return the pureed mixture to the pot. Fold in the coconut milk and continue to simmer until heated through or about 5 minutes longer.

Ladle into individual bowls and serve hot. Enjoy

59) FRENCH ORIGINAL ONION SOUP

Preparation Time: 1 hour 30 minutes		Servings: 4

Ingredients:

- 2 tbsp olive oil
- 2 large yellow onions, thinly sliced
- 2 thyme sprigs, chopped
- 2 rosemary sprigs, chopped
- 2 tsp balsamic vinegar
- 4 cups vegetable stock
- Sea salt and ground black pepper, to taste

Directions:

In a or Dutch oven, heat the olive oil over a moderate heat. Now, cook the onions with thyme, rosemary and 1 tsp of the sea salt for about 2 minutes.

Now, turn the heat to medium-low and continue cooking until the onions caramelize or about 50 minutes.

Add in the balsamic vinegar and continue to cook for a further 15 more. Add in the stock, salt and black pepper and continue simmering for 20 to 25 minutes.

Serve with toasted bread and enjoy

60) SUPER ROASTED CARROT SOUP

Preparation Time: 50 minutes		Servings: 4

Ingredients:

- ✓ 1 ½ pounds carrots
- ✓ 4 tbsp olive oil
- ✓ 1 yellow onion, chopped
- ✓ 2 cloves garlic, minced
- ✓ 1/3 tsp ground cumin
- ✓ Sea salt and white pepper, to taste
- ✓ 1/2 tsp turmeric powder
- ✓ 4 cups vegetable stock
- ✓ 2 tsp lemon juice
- ✓ 2 tbsp fresh cilantro, roughly chopped

Directions:

Start by preheating your oven to 400 degrees F. Place the carrots on a large parchment-lined baking sheet; toss the carrots with 2 tbsp of the olive oil.

Roast the carrots for about 35 minutes or until they've softened.

In a heavy-bottomed pot, heat the remaining 2 tbsp of the olive oil. Now, sauté the onion and garlic for about 3 minutes or until aromatic.

Add in the cumin, salt, pepper, turmeric, vegetable stock and roasted carrots. Continue to simmer for 12 minutes more.

Puree your soup with an immersion blender. Drizzle lemon juice over your soup and serve garnished with fresh cilantro leaves. Enjoy

61) ITALIAN-STYLE PENNE PASTA SALAD

Preparation Time: 15 minutes + chilling time		Servings: 3

Ingredients:

- ✓ 9 ounces penne pasta
- ✓ 9 ounces canned Cannellini bean, drained
- ✓ 1 small onion, thinly sliced
- ✓ 1/3 cup Niçoise olives, pitted and sliced
- ✓ 2 Italian peppers, sliced
- ✓ 1 cup cherry tomatoes, halved
- ✓ 3 cups arugula
- ✓ Dressing:
- ✓ 3 tbsp extra-virgin olive oil
- ✓ 1 tsp lemon zest
- ✓ 1 tsp garlic, minced
- ✓ 3 tbsp balsamic vinegar
- ✓ 1 tsp Italian herb mix
- ✓ Sea salt and ground black pepper, to taste

Directions:

Cook the penne pasta according to the package directions. Drain and rinse the pasta. Let it cool completely and then, transfer it to a salad bowl.

Then, add the beans, onion, olives, peppers, tomatoes and arugula to the salad bowl.

Mix all the dressing ingredients until everything is well incorporated. Dress your salad and serve well

62) SPECIAL CHANA CHAAT INDIAN SALAD

Preparation Time: 45 minutes + chilling time		Servings: 4

Ingredients:

- ✓ 1 pound dry chickpeas, soaked overnight
- ✓ 2 San Marzano tomatoes, diced
- ✓ 1 Persian cucumber, sliced
- ✓ 1 onion, chopped
- ✓ 1 bell pepper, seeded and thinly sliced
- ✓ 1 green chili, seeded and thinly sliced
- ✓ 2 handfuls baby spinach
- ✓ 1/2 tsp Kashmiri chili powder
- ✓ 4 curry leaves, chopped
- ✓ 1 tbsp chaat masala
- ✓ 2 tbsp fresh lemon juice, or to taste
- ✓ 4 tbsp olive oil
- ✓ 1 tsp agave syrup
- ✓ 1/2 tsp mustard seeds
- ✓ 1/2 tsp coriander seeds
- ✓ 2 tbsp sesame seeds, lightly toasted
- ✓ 2 tbsp fresh cilantro, roughly chopped

Directions:

Drain the chickpeas and transfer them to a large saucepan. Cover the chickpeas with water by 2 inches and bring it to a boil.

Immediately turn the heat to a simmer and continue to cook for approximately 40 minutes.

Toss the chickpeas with the tomatoes, cucumber, onion, peppers, spinach, chili powder, curry leaves and chaat masala.

In a small mixing dish, thoroughly combine the lemon juice, olive oil, agave syrup, mustard seeds and coriander seeds.

Garnish with sesame seeds and fresh cilantro. Enjoy

63) ORIGINAL TEMPEH AND NOODLE SALAD THAI-STYLE

Preparation Time: 45 minutes		Servings: 3

Ingredients:

- ✓ 6 ounces tempeh
- ✓ 4 tbsp rice vinegar
- ✓ 4 tbsp soy sauce
- ✓ 2 garlic cloves, minced
- ✓ 1 small-sized lime, freshly juiced
- ✓ 5 ounces rice noodles
- ✓ 1 carrot, julienned
- ✓ 1 shallot, chopped
- ✓ 3 handfuls Chinese cabbage, thinly sliced
- ✓ 3 handfuls kale, torn into pieces
- ✓ 1 bell pepper, seeded and thinly sliced
- ✓ 1 bird's eye chili, minced
- ✓ 1/4 cup peanut butter
- ✓ 2 tbsp agave syrup

Directions:

Place the tempeh, 2 tbsp of the rice vinegar, soy sauce, garlic and lime juice in a ceramic dish; let it marinate for about 40 minutes.

Meanwhile, cook the rice noodles according to the package directions. Drain your noodles and transfer them to a salad bowl.

Add the carrot, shallot, cabbage, kale and peppers to the salad bowl. Add in the peanut butter, the remaining 2 tbsp of the rice vinegar and agave syrup and toss to combine well.

Top with the marinated tempeh and serve immediately. Enjoy

64) TYPICAL CREAM OF BROCCOLI SOUP

Preparation Time: 35 minutes		Servings: 4

Ingredients:

- ✓ 2 tbsp olive oil
- ✓ 1 pound broccoli florets
- ✓ 1 onion, chopped
- ✓ 1 celery rib, chopped
- ✓ 1 parsnip, chopped
- ✓ 1 tsp garlic, chopped
- ✓ 3 cups vegetable broth
- ✓ 1/2 tsp dried dill
- ✓ 1/2 tsp dried oregano
- ✓ Sea salt and ground black pepper, to taste
- ✓ 2 tbsp flaxseed meal
- ✓ 1 cup full-fat coconut milk

Directions:

In a heavy-bottomed pot, heat the olive oil over medium-high heat. Now, sauté the broccoli onion, celery and parsnip for about 5 minutes, stirring periodically.

Add in the garlic and continue sautéing for 1 minute or until fragrant.

Then, stir in the vegetable broth, dill, oregano, salt and black pepper; bring to a boil. Immediately reduce the heat to a simmer and let it cook for about 20 minutes.

Puree the soup using an immersion blender until creamy and uniform.

Return the pureed mixture to the pot. Fold in the flaxseed meal and coconut milk; continue to simmer until heated through or about 5 minutes.

Ladle into four serving bowls and enjoy

65) EASY RAISIN MOROCCAN LENTIL SALAD

Preparation Time: 20 minutes + chilling time		Servings: 4

Ingredients:

- ✓ 1 cup red lentils, rinsed
- ✓ 1 large carrot, julienned
- ✓ 1 Persian cucumber, thinly sliced
- ✓ 1 sweet onion, chopped
- ✓ 1/2 cup golden raisins
- ✓ 1/4 cup fresh mint, snipped
- ✓ 1/4 cup fresh basil, snipped
- ✓ 1/4 cup extra-virgin olive oil
- ✓ 1/4 cup lemon juice, freshly squeezed
- ✓ 1 tsp grated lemon peel
- ✓ 1/2 tsp fresh ginger root, peeled and minced
- ✓ 1/2 tsp granulated garlic
- ✓ 1 tsp ground allspice
- ✓ Sea salt and ground black pepper, to taste

Directions:

In a large-sized saucepan, bring 3 cups of the water and 1 cup of the lentils to a boil.

Immediately turn the heat to a simmer and continue to cook your lentils for a further 15 to 17 minutes or until they've softened but are not mushy yet. Drain and let it cool completely.

Transfer the lentils to a salad bowl; add in the carrot, cucumber and sweet onion. Then, add the raisins, mint and basil to your salad.

In a small mixing dish, whisk the olive oil, lemon juice, lemon peel, ginger, granulated garlic, allspice, salt and black pepper.

Dress your salad and serve well-chilled. Enjoy

66) RICH CHICKPEA AND ASPARAGUS SALAD

Preparation Time: 10 minutes + chilling time | | **Servings: 5**

Ingredients:

- ✓ 1 ¼ pounds asparagus, trimmed and cut into bite-sized pieces
- ✓ 5 ounces canned chickpeas, drained and rinsed
- ✓ 1 chipotle pepper, seeded and chopped
- ✓ 1 Italian pepper, seeded and chopped
- ✓ 1/4 cup fresh basil leaves, chopped
- ✓ 1/4 cup fresh parsley leaves, chopped

- ✓ 2 tbsp fresh mint leaves
- ✓ 2 tbsp fresh chives, chopped
- ✓ 1 tsp garlic, minced
- ✓ 1/4 cup extra-virgin olive oil
- ✓ 1 tbsp balsamic vinegar
- ✓ 1 tbsp fresh lime juice
- ✓ 2 tbsp soy sauce
- ✓ 1/4 tsp ground allspice
- ✓ 1/4 tsp ground cumin
- ✓ Sea salt and freshly cracked peppercorns, to taste

Directions:

Bring a large pot of salted water with the asparagus to a boil; let it cook for 2 minutes; drain and rinse.

Transfer the asparagus to a salad bowl.

Toss the asparagus with the chickpeas, peppers, herbs, garlic, olive oil, vinegar, lime juice, soy sauce and spices.

Toss to combine and serve immediately. Enjoy

67) OLD-FASHIONED GREEK GREEN BEAN SALAD

Preparation Time: 10 minutes + chilling time | | **Servings: 4**

Ingredients:

- ✓ 1 ½ pounds green beans, trimmed
- ✓ 1/2 cup scallions, chopped
- ✓ 1 tsp garlic, minced
- ✓ 1 Persian cucumber, sliced
- ✓ 2 cups grape tomatoes, halved
- ✓ 1/4 cup olive oil

- ✓ 1 tsp deli mustard
- ✓ 2 tbsp tamari sauce
- ✓ 2 tbsp lemon juice
- ✓ 1 tbsp apple cider vinegar
- ✓ 1/4 tsp cumin powder
- ✓ 1/2 tsp dried thyme
- ✓ Sea salt and ground black pepper, to taste

Directions:

Boil the green beans in a large saucepan of salted water until they are just tender or about 2 minutes.

Drain and let the beans cool completely; then, transfer them to a salad bowl. Toss the beans with the remaining ingredients.

Enjoy

68) AUTUMN BEAN SOUP

Preparation Time: 25 minutes | | **Servings: 4**

Ingredients:

- ✓ 1 tbsp olive oil
- ✓ 2 tbsp shallots, chopped
- ✓ 1 carrot, chopped
- ✓ 1 parsnip, chopped
- ✓ 1 celery stalk, chopped

- ✓ 1 tsp fresh garlic, minced
- ✓ 4 cups vegetable broth
- ✓ 2 bay leaves
- ✓ 1 rosemary sprig, chopped
- ✓ 16 ounces canned navy beans
- ✓ Flaky sea salt and ground black pepper, to taste

Directions:

In a heavy-bottomed pot, heat the olive over medium-high heat. Now, sauté the shallots, carrot, parsnip and celery for approximately 3 minutes or until the vegetables are just tender.

Add in the garlic and continue to sauté for 1 minute or until aromatic.

Then, add in the vegetable broth, bay leaves and rosemary and bring to a boil. Immediately reduce the heat to a simmer and let it cook for 10 minutes.

Fold in the navy beans and continue to simmer for about 5 minutes longer until everything is thoroughly heated. Season with salt and black pepper to taste.

Ladle into individual bowls, discard the bay leaves and serve hot. Enjoy

69) ITALIAN CREAM MUSHROOMS SOUP

Preparation Time: 15 minutes		Servings: 3

Ingredients:

- ✓ 3 tbsp vegan butter
- ✓ 1 white onion, chopped
- ✓ 1 red bell pepper, chopped
- ✓ 1/2 tsp garlic, pressed
- ✓ 3 cups Cremini mushrooms, chopped
- ✓ 2 tbsp almond flour
- ✓ 3 cups water
- ✓ 1 tsp Italian herb mix
- ✓ Sea salt and ground black pepper, to taste
- ✓ 1 heaping tbsp fresh chives, roughly chopped

Directions:

In a stockpot, melt the vegan butter over medium-high heat. Once hot, sauté the onion and pepper for about 3 minutes until they have softened.

Add in the garlic and Cremini mushrooms and continue sautéing until the mushrooms have softened. Sprinkle almond meal over the mushrooms and continue to cook for 1 minute or so.

Add in the remaining ingredients. Let it simmer, covered and continue to cook for 5 to 6 minutes more until the liquid has thickened slightly.

Ladle into three soup bowls and garnish with fresh chives. Enjoy

70) TASTY ROASTED BASIL AND TOMATO SOUP

Preparation Time: 60 minutes		Servings: 4

Ingredients:

- ✓ 2 lb tomatoes, halved
- ✓ 2 tsp garlic powder
- ✓ 3 tbsp olive oil
- ✓ 1 tbsp balsamic vinegar
- ✓ Salt and black pepper to taste
- ✓ 4 shallots, chopped
- ✓ 2 cups vegetable broth
- ✓ ½ cup basil leaves, chopped

Directions:

Preheat oven to 450 F.

In a bowl, mix tomatoes, garlic, 2 tbsp of oil, vinegar, salt, and pepper. Arrange the tomatoes onto a baking dish. Sprinkle with some olive oil, garlic powder, balsamic vinegar, salt, and pepper. Bake for 30 minutes until the tomatoes get dark brown color. Take out from the oven; reserve.

Heat the remaining oil in a pot over medium heat. Place the shallots and cook for 3 minutes, stirring often. Add in roasted tomatoes and broth. Bring to a boil, then lower the heat and simmer for 10 minutes. Transfer to a food processor and blitz the soup until smooth. Serve topped with basil

71) SPECIAL UNDER PRESSURE COOKER GREEN ONION AND POTATO SOUP

Preparation Time: 25 minutes		Servings: 5

Ingredients:

- ✓ 3 green onions, chopped
- ✓ 4 garlic cloves, minced
- ✓ 1 tbsp olive oil
- ✓ 6 russet potatoes, chopped
- ✓ ½ (13.5-oz) can coconut milk
- ✓ 5 cups vegetable broth
- ✓ Salt and black pepper to taste

Directions:

Set your IP to Sauté. Place in green onions, garlic, and olive oil. Cook for 3 minutes until softened. Add in potatoes, coconut milk, broth, and salt. Lock the lid in place, set time to 6 minutes on High. Once ready, perform a natural pressure release for 10 minutes. Allow cooling for a few minutes. Using an immersion blender, blitz the soup until smooth. Serve

72) EASY AND QUICK BELL PEPPER AND MUSHROOM SOUP

Preparation Time: 45 minutes		Servings: 6

Ingredients:

- ✓ 3 tbsp olive oil
- ✓ 1 onion, chopped
- ✓ 1 large carrot, chopped
- ✓ 1 lb mixed bell peppers, chopped
- ✓ 1 cup cremini mushrooms, quartered
- ✓ 1 cup white mushrooms, quartered
- ✓ 6 cups vegetable broth
- ✓ ¼ cup chopped fresh parsley
- ✓ 1 tsp minced fresh thyme
- ✓ Salt and black pepper to taste

Directions:

Heat the oil in a pot over medium heat. Place onion, carrot, and celery and cook for 5 minutes. Add in bell peppers and broth and stir. Bring to a boil, lower the heat, and simmer for 20 minutes. Adjust the seasoning with salt and black pepper. Serve in soup bowls topped with parsley and thyme

73) SUPER INDIAN-STYLE TURNIP SOUP

Preparation Time: 30 minutes		Servings: 4

Ingredients:

- ✓ 2 tbsp olive oil
- ✓ 1 onion, chopped
- ✓ 3/4 pound turnip, trimmed and sliced
- ✓ 1/4 pound carrot, trimmed and sliced
- ✓ 1/4 cup parsnip, trimmed and sliced
- ✓ 1 tbsp ginger-garlic paste
- ✓ 3 cups water
- ✓ 1/2 tsp coriander seeds
- ✓ 1/2 tsp celery seeds
- ✓ 1/2 tsp fennel seeds
- ✓ 1 tsp curry powder
- ✓ Sea salt and ground black pepper
- ✓ 1 tbsp bouillon granules
- ✓ 1/2 cup raw cashews, soaked
- ✓ 1 cup water, divided
- ✓ 1 tbsp lemon juice

Directions:

In a heavy-bottomed pot, heat the olive oil over medium-high heat. Now, sauté the onion, turnip, carrot and parsnip for about 5 minutes, stirring periodically.

Add in the ginger-garlic paste and continue sautéing for 1 minute or until fragrant.

Then, stir in the water, coriander seeds, celery seeds, fennel seeds, curry powder, salt, black pepper and bouillon granules; bring to a boil. Immediately reduce the heat to a simmer and let it cook for about 20 to 22 minutes.

Puree the soup using an immersion blender until creamy and uniform.

Drain the cashews and add them to the bowl of your blender or food processor; add in the water, lemon juice and salt to taste. Blend into a cream.

Return the pureed mixture to the pot. Fold in the cashew cream and continue simmering until heated through or about 5 minutes longer.

Ladle into serving bowls and serve hot. Enjoy

74) SPRING ROOT VEGETABLE SOUP

Preparation Time: 40 minutes		Servings: 4

Ingredients:

- ✓ 4 tbsp avocado oil
- ✓ 1 large leek, sliced
- ✓ 2 carrots, diced
- ✓ 2 parsnips, diced
- ✓ 2 cups turnip, diced
- ✓ 2 celery stalks, diced
- ✓ 1 pound sweet potatoes, diced
- ✓ 1 tsp ginger-garlic paste
- ✓ 1 habanero pepper, seeded and chopped
- ✓ 1/2 tsp caraway seeds
- ✓ 1/2 tsp fennel seeds
- ✓ 2 bay leaves
- ✓ Sea salt and ground black pepper, to season
- ✓ 1 tsp cayenne pepper
- ✓ 4 cups vegetable broth
- ✓ 4 tbsp tahini

Directions:

In a stockpot, heat the oil over medium-high heat. Now, sauté the leeks, carrots, parsnip, turnip, celery and sweet potatoes for about 5 minutes, stirring periodically.

Add in the ginger-garlic paste and habanero peppers and continue sautéing for 1 minute or until fragrant.

Then, stir in the caraway seeds, fennel seeds, bay leaves, salt, black pepper, cayenne pepper and vegetable broth; bring to a boil. Immediately turn the heat to a simmer and let it cook for approximately 25 minutes.

Puree the soup using an immersion blender until creamy and uniform.

Return the pureed mixture to the pot. Fold in the tahini and continue to simmer until heated through or about 5 minutes longer.

Ladle into individual bowls and serve hot. Enjoy

75) GREEK-STYLE SALAD

Preparation Time: 10 minutes		Servings: 2

Ingredients:

- ✓ ½ yellow bell pepper, cut into pieces
- ✓ 3 tomatoes cut into bite-size pieces
- ✓ ½ cucumber, cut into bite-size pieces
- ✓ ½ red onion, peeled and sliced
- ✓ ½ cup tofu cheese, cut into squares
- ✓ 10 Kalamata olives, pitted
- ✓ ½ tbsp red wine vinegar
- ✓ 4 tbsp olive oil
- ✓ 2 tsp dried oregano

Directions:

Pour the bell pepper, tomatoes, cucumber, red onion, tofu cheese, and olives into a salad bowl. Drizzle the red wine vinegar and olive oil over the vegetables. Season with salt, black pepper, and oregano, and toss the salad with two spoons. Share the salad into two bowls and serve immediately

76) SPECIAL SQUASH SALAD

Preparation Time: 20 minutes		Servings: 4

Ingredients:

- ✓ 2 lb green squash, cubed
- ✓ 2 tbsp plant butter
- ✓ Salt and black pepper to taste
- ✓ 3 oz fennel, sliced
- ✓ 2 oz chopped green onions
- ✓ 1 cup tofu mayonnaise
- ✓ 2 tbsp fresh chives, finely chopped
- ✓ A pinch of mustard powder
- ✓ Chopped dill to garnish

Directions:

Put a pan over medium heat and melt plant butter. Fry in squash cubes until slightly softened but not browned, about 7 minutes. Allow the squash to cool. In a salad bowl, mix the cooled squash, fennel slices, green onions, tofu mayonnaise, chives, and mustard powder. Garnish with dill and serve

77) SUPER BEET TOFU SALAD

Preparation Time: 50 minutes		Servings: 4

Ingredients:

- ✓ 8 oz red beets
- ✓ 2 oz tofu, chopped into little bits
- ✓ 2 tbsp plant butter
- ✓ ½ red onion
- ✓ 1 cup tofu mayonnaise
- ✓ 1 small romaine lettuce, torn
- ✓ Freshly chopped chives
- ✓ Salt and black pepper to taste

Directions:

Put beets in a pot, cover with water, and bring to a boil for 40 minutes. Melt plant butter in a non-stick pan over medium heat and fry tofu until browned. Set aside to cool. When the bits are ready, drain through a colander and allow cooling. Slip the skin off after and slice them. In a salad bowl, combine the beets, tofu, red onions, lettuce, salt, pepper, and tofu mayonnaise and mix until the vegetables are adequately coated with the mayonnaise. Garnish with chives and serve

78) EXOTIC MANGO RICE SALAD WITH LIME DRESSING

Preparation Time: 15 minutes | | **Servings:** 4

Ingredients:

- ✓ 3 ½ cups cooked brown rice
- ✓ ½ cup chopped roasted peanuts
- ✓ ½ cup sliced mango
- ✓ 4 green onions, chopped
- ✓ 3 tbsp fresh lime juice
- ✓ 2 tsp agave nectar
- ✓ 1 tsp grated fresh ginger
- ✓ 1/3 cup grapeseed oil
- ✓ Salt and black pepper to taste

Directions:

n a bowl, mix the rice, peanuts, mango, and green onions. Set aside. In another bowl, whisk the lime juice, agave nectar, and ginger. Add in oil, salt and pepper, stir to combine. Pour over the rice bowl and toss to coat. Serve immediately

79) ORIGINAL PASTA SALAD WITH CANNELLINI BEANS

Preparation Time: 35 minutes | | **Servings:** 4

Ingredients:

- ✓ 2 ½ cups whole-wheat bow tie pasta
- ✓ 1 tbsp olive oil
- ✓ 1 medium zucchini, sliced
- ✓ 2 garlic cloves, minced
- ✓ 2 large tomatoes, chopped
- ✓ 1 (15 oz) can cannellini beans
- ✓ 1 (2 ¼ oz) can green olives, sliced
- ✓ ½ cup crumbled tofu cheese

Directions:

Cook the pasta until al dente, 10 minutes. Drain and set aside. Heat olive oil in a skillet and sauté zucchini and garlic for 4 minutes. Stir in tomatoes, beans, and olives. Cook until the tomatoes soften, 10 minutes. Mix in pasta. Allow warming for 1 minute. Stir in tofu cheese and serve warm

80) MEXICAN BEAN AND FARRO SALAD

Preparation Time: 20 minutes | | **Servings:** 4

Ingredients:

- ✓ 1 (14-oz) can black beans
- ✓ 1 cup corn kernels
- ✓ ¼ cup fresh cilantro, chopped
- ✓ Zest and juice of 1 lime
- ✓ 3 tsp chili powder
- ✓ Sea salt and black pepper to taste
- ✓ 1 ½ cups cherry tomatoes, halved
- ✓ 1 red bell pepper, chopped
- ✓ 2 scallions, chopped
- ✓ 4 large whole-grain tortillas
- ✓ 2 tsp olive oil
- ✓ 1 tbsp oregano
- ✓ 1 tsp cayenne pepper
- ✓ 4 cups watercress and arugula mix
- ✓ ¾ cup cooked faro
- ✓ ¼ cup chopped avocado
- ✓ ¼ cup mango salsa

Directions:

Combine black beans, corn, cilantro, lime juice, lime zest, chili powder, salt, pepper, cherry tomatoes, bell peppers, and scallions in a bowl. Set aside. Brush the tortillas with olive oil and season with salt, pepper, oregano, and cayenne pepper. Slice into 8 pieces. Line with parchment paper a baking sheet. Arrange tortilla pieces and bake for 3-5 minutes until browned. On a serving platter, put the watercress and arugula mix, top with faro, bean mixture, avocado, and sprinkle with mango salsa all over to serve

81) TASTY ORANGE AND KALE SALAD

Preparation Time: 10 minutes		Servings: 4

Ingredients:

- ✓ 2 tbsp Dijon mustard
- ✓ 2 tbsp olive oil
- ✓ ¼ cup fresh orange juice
- ✓ 1 tsp agave nectar
- ✓ 2 tbsp minced fresh parsley
- ✓ 1 tbsp minced green onions
- ✓ 4 cups fresh kale, chopped
- ✓ 1 orange, peeled and segmented
- ✓ ½ red onion, sliced paper-thin

Directions:

In a food processor, place the mustard, oil, orange juice, agave nectar, salt, pepper, parsley, and green onions. Blend until smooth. Set aside. In a bowl, combine the kale, orange, and onion. Pour over the dressing and toss to coat. Serve

82) AFRICAN-STYLE ZUCCHINI SALAD

Preparation Time: 20 minutes		Servings: 2

Ingredients:

- ✓ 1 lemon, half zested and juiced, half cut into wedges
- ✓ 1 tsp olive oil 1 zucchini, chopped
- ✓ ½ tsp ground cumin
- ✓ ½ tsp ground ginger
- ✓ ¼ tsp turmeric
- ✓ ¼ tsp ground nutmeg
- ✓ A pinch of salt
- ✓ 2 tbsp capers
- ✓ 1 tbsp chopped green olives
- ✓ 1 garlic clove, pressed
- ✓ 2 tbsp fresh mint, finely chopped
- ✓ 2 cups spinach, chopped

Directions:

Warm olive oil in a skillet over medium heat. Place the zucchini and sauté for 10 minutes. Stir in cumin, ginger, turmeric, nutmeg, and salt. Pour in lemon zest, lemon juice, capers, garlic, and mint, cook for 2 minutes more. Divide the spinach between serving plates and top with the zucchini mixture. Garnish with lemon wedges and olives

83) EASY TANGY NUTTY BRUSSEL SPROUT SALAD

Preparation Time: 20 minutes		Servings: 4

Ingredients:

- ✓ 1 lb Brussels sprouts, grated
- ✓ 1 lemon, juiced and zested
- ✓ ½ cup olive oil
- ✓ 1 tbsp plant butter
- ✓ 1 tsp chili paste
- ✓ 2 oz pecans
- ✓ 1 oz pumpkin seeds
- ✓ 1 oz sunflower seeds
- ✓ ½ tsp cumin powder

Directions:

Put Brussels sprouts in a salad bowl. In a small bowl, mix lemon juice, zest, olive oil, salt, and pepper, and drizzle the dressing over the Brussels sprouts. Toss and allow the vegetable to marinate for 10 minutes. Melt plant butter in a pan. Stir in chili paste and toss the pecans, pumpkin seeds, sunflower seeds, cumin powder, and salt in the chili butter. Sauté on low heat for 3-4 minutes just to heat the nuts. Allow cooling. Pour the nuts and seeds mix in the salad bowl, toss, and serve

84) ITALIAN MUSHROOM SOUP OF MEDLEY

Preparation Time: 40 minutes		Servings: 4

Ingredients:

- ✓ 4 oz unsalted plant butter
- ✓ 1 small onion, finely chopped
- ✓ 1 clove garlic, minced
- ✓ 5 oz button mushrooms, chopped
- ✓ 5 oz cremini mushrooms, chopped
- ✓ 5 oz shiitake mushrooms, chopped
- ✓ ½ lb celery root, chopped
- ✓ ½ tsp dried rosemary
- ✓ 1 vegetable stock cube, crushed
- ✓ 1 tbsp plain vinegar
- ✓ 1 cup coconut cream
- ✓ 4 – 6 leaves basil, chopped

Directions:

- ❖ Place a saucepan over medium-high heat, add the plant butter to melt, then sauté the onion, garlic, mushrooms, and celery root in the butter until golden brown and fragrant, about 6 minutes. Fetch out some mushrooms and reserve for garnishing. Add the rosemary, 3 cups of water, stock cube, and vinegar. Stir the mixture and bring it to a boil for 6 minutes. After, reduce the heat and simmer the soup for 15 minutes or until the celery is soft.
- ❖ Mix in the coconut cream and puree the ingredients using an immersion blender. Simmer for 2 minutes. Spoon the soup into serving bowls, garnish with the reserved mushrooms and basil. Serve

85) MEDITERRANEAN DILL CAULIFLOWER SOUP

Preparation Time: 26 minutes		Servings: 4

Ingredients:

- ✓ 2 tbsp coconut oil
- ✓ ½ lb celery root, trimmed
- ✓ 1 garlic clove
- ✓ 1 medium white onion
- ✓ ¼ cup fresh dill, roughly chopped
- ✓ 1 tsp cumin powder
- ✓ ¼ tsp nutmeg powder
- ✓ 1 head cauliflower, cut into florets
- ✓ 3 ½ cups seasoned vegetable stock
- ✓ 5 oz plant butter
- ✓ Juice from 1 lemon
- ✓ ¼ cup coconut whipping cream

Directions:

- ❖ Set a pot over medium heat, add the coconut oil and allow heating until no longer shimmering.
- ❖ Add the celery root, garlic clove, and onion; sauté the vegetables until fragrant and soft, about 5 minutes. Stir in the dill, cumin, and nutmeg, and fry further for 1 minute. Mix in the cauliflower florets and vegetable stock. Bring the soup to a boil for 12 to 15 minutes or until the cauliflower is soft. Turn the heat off. Add the plant butter and lemon juice. Puree the ingredients with an immersion blender until smooth. Mix in coconut whipping cream and season the soup with salt and black pepper. Serve warm

86) SPECIAL FENNEL BROCCOLI SOUP

Preparation Time: 25 minutes		Servings: 4

Ingredients:

- ✓ 1 fennel bulb, chopped
- ✓ 10 oz broccoli, cut into florets
- ✓ 3 cups vegetable stock
- ✓ Salt and black pepper to taste
- ✓ 1 garlic clove
- ✓ 1 cup cashew cream cheese
- ✓ 3 oz plant butter
- ✓ ½ cup chopped fresh oregano

Directions:

- ❖ Put the fennel and broccoli into a pot, and cover with the vegetable stock. Bring the ingredients to a boil over medium heat until the vegetables are soft, about 10 minutes. Season the liquid with salt and black pepper, and drop in the garlic. Simmer the soup for 5 to 7 minutes and turn the heat off.
- ❖ Pour the cream cheese, plant butter, and oregano into the soup; puree the ingredients with an immersion blender until completely smooth. Adjust the taste with salt and black pepper. Spoon the soup into serving bowls and serve

87) EASY BEAN SOUP ASIAN-STYLE

Preparation Time: 55 minutes		Servings: 4

Ingredients:

- ✓ 1 cup canned cannellini beans
- ✓ 2 tsp curry powder
- ✓ 2 tsp olive oil
- ✓ 1 red onion, diced
- ✓ 1 tbsp minced fresh ginger
- ✓ 2 cubed sweet potatoes
- ✓ 1 cup sliced zucchini
- ✓ Salt and black pepper to taste
- ✓ 4 cups vegetable stock
- ✓ 1 bunch spinach, chopped
- ✓ Toasted sesame seeds

Directions:

- ❖ Mix the beans with 1 tsp of curry powder until well combined. Warm the oil in a pot over medium heat. Place the onion and ginger and cook for 5 minutes until soft. Add in sweet potatoes and cook for 10 minutes. Put in zucchini and cook for 5 minutes. Season with the remaining curry, pepper, and salt.
- ❖ Pour in the stock and bring to a boil. Lower the heat and simmer for 25 minutes. Stir in beans and spinach. Cook until the spinach wilts and remove from the heat. Garnish with sesame seeds to serve

88) TORTILLA MEXICAN-STYLE SOUP

Preparation Time: 40 minutes		Servings: 4

Ingredients:

- ✓ 1 (14.5-oz) can diced tomatoes
- ✓ 1 (4-oz) can green chiles, chopped
- ✓ 2 tbsp olive oil
- ✓ 1 cup canned sweet corn
- ✓ 1 red onion, chopped
- ✓ 2 garlic cloves, minced
- ✓ 2 jalapeño peppers, sliced
- ✓ 4 cups vegetable broth
- ✓ 8 oz seitan, cut into ¼-inch strips
- ✓ Salt and black pepper to taste
- ✓ ¼ cup chopped fresh cilantro
- ✓ 3 tbsp fresh lime juice
- ✓ 4 corn tortillas, cut into strips
- ✓ 1 ripe avocado, chopped

Directions:

- ❖ Preheat oven to 350 F. Heat the oil in a pot over medium heat. Place sweet corn, garlic, jalapeño, and onion and cook for 5 minutes. Stir in broth, seitan, tomatoes, canned chiles, salt, and pepper. Bring to a boil, then lower the heat and simmer for 20 minutes. Put in the cilantro and lime juice, stir. Adjust the seasoning.
- ❖ Meanwhile, arrange the tortilla strips on a baking sheet and bake for 8 minutes until crisp. Serve the soup into bowls and top with tortilla strips and avocado

89) HOT BEAN SPICY SOUP

Preparation Time: 40 minutes		Servings: 4

Ingredients:

- ✓ 2 tbsp olive oil
- ✓ 1 medium onion, chopped
- ✓ 2 large garlic cloves, minced
- ✓ 1 carrot, chopped
- ✓ 1 (15.5-oz) can cannellini beans, drained
- ✓ 5 cups vegetable broth
- ✓ ¼ tsp crushed red pepper
- ✓ Salt and black pepper to taste
- ✓ 3 cups chopped baby spinach

Directions:

- ❖ Heat oil in a pot over medium heat. Place in carrot, onion, and garlic and cook for 3 minutes. Put in beans, broth, red pepper, salt, and black pepper and stir. Bring to a boil, then lower the heat and simmer for 25 minutes. Stir in baby spinach and cook for 5 minutes until the spinach wilts. Serve warm

90) SPECIAL MUSHROOM RICE WINE SOUP

Preparation Time: 25 minutes		Servings: 4

Ingredients:

- ✓ 2 tbsp olive oil
- ✓ 4 green onions, chopped
- ✓ 1 carrot, chopped
- ✓ 8 oz shiitake mushrooms, sliced
- ✓ 3 tbsp rice wine
- ✓ 2 tbsp soy sauce
- ✓ 4 cups vegetable broth
- ✓ Salt and black pepper to taste
- ✓ 2 tbsp parsley, chopped

Directions:

- ❖ Heat the oil in a pot over medium heat. Place the green onions and carrot and cook for 5 minutes.
- ❖ Stir in mushrooms, rice wine, soy sauce, broth, salt, and pepper. Bring to a boil, then lower the heat and simmer for 15 minutes. Top with parsley and serve warm

91) TASTY BEAN TANGY TOMATO SOUP

Preparation Time: 30 minutes | | **Servings:** 5

Ingredients:

- ✓ 2 tsp olive oil
- ✓ 1 onion, chopped
- ✓ 2 garlic cloves, minced
- ✓ 1 cup mushrooms, chopped
- ✓ Sea salt to taste
- ✓ 1 tbsp dried basil
- ✓ ½ tbsp dried oregano
- ✓ 1 (19-oz) can diced tomatoes
- ✓ 1 (14-oz) can kidney beans, drained
- ✓ 5 cups water
- ✓ 2 cups chopped mustard greens

Directions:

- ❖ Heat the oil in a pot over medium heat. Place in the onion, garlic, mushrooms, and salt and cook for 5 minutes. Stir in basil and oregano, tomatoes, and beans. Pour in water and stir. Simmer for 20 minutes and add in mustard greens; cook for 5 minutes until greens soften. Serve immediately

92) EASY SPINACH AND POTATO SOUP

Preparation Time: 55 minutes | | **Servings:** 4

Ingredients:

- ✓ 2 tbsp olive oil
- ✓ 1 onion, chopped
- ✓ 2 garlic cloves, minced
- ✓ 4 cups vegetable broth
- ✓ 2 russet potatoes, cubed
- ✓ ½ tsp dried oregano
- ✓ ¼ tsp crushed red pepper
- ✓ 1 bay leaf
- ✓ Salt to taste
- ✓ 4 cups chopped spinach
- ✓ 1 cup green lentils, rinsed

Directions:

- ❖ Warm the oil in a pot over medium heat. Place the onion and garlic and cook covered for 5 minutes. Stir in broth, potatoes, oregano, red pepper, bay leaf, lentils, and salt. Bring to a boil, then lower the heat and simmer uncovered for 30 minutes. Add in spinach and cook for another 5 minutes. Discard the bay leaf and serve immediately

93) MEXICAN BEAN TURMERIC SOUP

Preparation Time: 50 minutes | | **Servings:** 6

Ingredients:

- ✓ 3 tbsp olive oil
- ✓ 1 onion, chopped
- ✓ 2 carrots, chopped
- ✓ 1 sweet potato, chopped
- ✓ 1 yellow bell pepper, chopped
- ✓ 2 garlic cloves, minced
- ✓ 4 tomatoes, chopped
- ✓ 6 cups vegetable broth
- ✓ 1 bay leaf
- ✓ Salt to taste
- ✓ 1 tsp ground cayenne pepper
- ✓ 1 (15.5-oz) can white beans, drained
- ✓ ⅓ cup whole-wheat pasta
- ✓ ¼ tsp turmeric

Directions:

- ❖ Heat the oil in a pot over medium heat. Place onion, carrots, sweet potato, bell pepper, and garlic. Cook for 5 minutes. Add in tomatoes, broth, bay leaf, salt, and cayenne pepper. Stir and bring to a boil. Lower the heat and simmer for 10 minutes. Put in white beans and simmer for 15 more minutes.
- ❖ Cook the pasta in a pot with boiling salted water and turmeric for 8-10 minutes, until pasta is al dente. Strain and transfer to the soup. Discard the bay leaf. Spoon into a bowl and serve

94) TROPICAL COCONUT ARUGULA SOUP

Preparation Time: 30 minutes | | **Servings: 4**

Ingredients:

- ✓ 1 tsp coconut oil
- ✓ 1 onion, diced
- ✓ 2 cups green beans
- ✓ 4 cups water
- ✓ 1 cup arugula, chopped
- ✓ 1 tbsp fresh mint, chopped
- ✓ Sea salt and black pepper to taste
- ✓ ¾ cup coconut milk

Directions:

- ❖ Place a pot over medium heat and heat the coconut oil. Add in the onion and sauté for 5 minutes. Pour in green beans and water. Bring to a boil, lower the heat and stir in arugula, mint, salt, and pepper. Simmer for 10 minutes. Stir in coconut milk. Transfer to a food processor and blitz the soup until smooth. Serve

95) AUTHENTIC LENTIL SOUP WITH SWISS CHARD

Preparation Time: 25 minutes | | **Servings: 5**

Ingredients:

- ✓ 2 tbsp olive oil
- ✓ 1 white onion, chopped
- ✓ 1 tsp garlic, minced
- ✓ 2 large carrots, chopped
- ✓ 1 parsnip, chopped
- ✓ 2 stalks celery, chopped
- ✓ 2 bay leaves
- ✓ 1/2 tsp dried thyme
- ✓ 1/4 tsp ground cumin
- ✓ 5 cups roasted vegetable broth
- ✓ 1 ¼ cups brown lentils, soaked overnight and rinsed
- ✓ 2 cups Swiss chard, torn into pieces

Directions:

- ❖ In a heavy-bottomed pot, heat the olive oil over a moderate heat. Now, sauté the vegetables along with the spices for about 3 minutes until they are just tender.
- ❖ Add in the vegetable broth and lentils, bringing it to a boil. Immediately turn the heat to a simmer and add in the bay leaves. Let it cook for about 15 minutes or until lentils are tender.
- ❖ Add in the Swiss chard, cover and let it simmer for 5 minutes more or until the chard wilts.
- ❖ Serve in individual bowls and enjoy

96) AUTUMN SPICY FARRO SOUP

Preparation Time: 30 minutes | | **Servings: 4**

Ingredients:

- ✓ 2 tbsp olive oil
- ✓ 1 medium-sized leek, chopped
- ✓ 1 medium-sized turnip, sliced
- ✓ 2 Italian peppers, seeded and chopped
- ✓ 1 jalapeno pepper, minced
- ✓ 2 potatoes, peeled and diced
- ✓ 4 cups vegetable broth
- ✓ 1 cup farro, rinsed
- ✓ 1/2 tsp granulated garlic
- ✓ 1/2 tsp turmeric powder
- ✓ 1 bay laurel
- ✓ 2 cups spinach, turn into pieces

Directions:

- ❖ In a heavy-bottomed pot, heat the olive oil over a moderate heat. Now, sauté the leek, turnip, peppers and potatoes for about 5 minutes until they are crisp-tender.
- ❖ Add in the vegetable broth, farro, granulated garlic, turmeric and bay laurel; bring it to a boil.
- ❖ Immediately turn the heat to a simmer. Let it cook for about 25 minutes or until farro and potatoes have softened.
- ❖ Add in the spinach and remove the pot from the heat; let the spinach sit in the residual heat until it wilts. Enjoy

97) ALL COLORED CHICKPEA SALAD

Preparation Time: 30 minutes		**Servings: 4**

Ingredients:

- ✓ 16 ounces canned chickpeas, drained
- ✓ 1 medium avocado, sliced
- ✓ 1 bell pepper, seeded and sliced
- ✓ 1 large tomato, sliced
- ✓ 2 cucumber, diced
- ✓ 1 red onion, sliced
- ✓ 1/2 tsp garlic, minced
- ✓ 1/4 cup fresh parsley, chopped
- ✓ 1/4 cup olive oil
- ✓ 2 tbsp apple cider vinegar
- ✓ 1/2 lime, freshly squeezed
- ✓ Sea salt and ground black pepper, to taste

Directions:

- ❖ Toss all the ingredients in a salad bowl.
- ❖ Place the salad in your refrigerator for about 1 hour before serving.
- ❖ Enjoy

98) MEDITERRANEAN-STYLE LENTIL SALAD

Preparation Time: 20 minutes + chilling time		**Servings: 5**

Ingredients:

- ✓ 1 ½ cups red lentil, rinsed
- ✓ 1 tsp deli mustard
- ✓ 1/2 lemon, freshly squeezed
- ✓ 2 tbsp tamari sauce
- ✓ 2 scallion stalks, chopped
- ✓ 1/4 cup extra-virgin olive oil
- ✓ 2 garlic cloves, minced
- ✓ 1 cup butterhead lettuce, torn into pieces
- ✓ 2 tbsp fresh parsley, chopped
- ✓ 2 tbsp fresh cilantro, chopped
- ✓ 1 tsp fresh basil
- ✓ 1 tsp fresh oregano
- ✓ 1 ½ cups cherry tomatoes, halved
- ✓ 3 ounces Kalamata olives, pitted and halved

Directions:

- ❖ In a large-sized saucepan, bring 4 ½ cups of the water and the red lentils to a boil.
- ❖ Immediately turn the heat to a simmer and continue to cook your lentils for about 15 minutes or until tender. Drain and let it cool completely.
- ❖ Transfer the lentils to a salad bowl; toss the lentils with the remaining ingredients until well combined.
- ❖ Serve chilled or at room temperature. Enjoy

99) DELICIOUS ROASTED AVOCADO AND ASPARAGUS SALAD

Preparation Time: 20 minutes + chilling time		**Servings: 4**

Ingredients:

- ✓ 1 pound asparagus, trimmed, cut into bite-sized pieces
- ✓ 1 white onion, chopped
- ✓ 2 garlic cloves, minced
- ✓ 1 Roma tomato, sliced
- ✓ 1/4 cup olive oil
- ✓ 1/4 cup balsamic vinegar
- ✓ 1 tbsp stone-ground mustard
- ✓ 2 tbsp fresh parsley, chopped
- ✓ 1 tbsp fresh cilantro, chopped
- ✓ 1 tbsp fresh basil, chopped
- ✓ Sea salt and ground black pepper, to taste
- ✓ 1 small avocado, pitted and diced
- ✓ 1/2 cup pine nuts, roughly chopped

Directions:

- ❖ Begin by preheating your oven to 420 degrees F.
- ❖ Toss the asparagus with 1 tbsp of the olive oil and arrange them on a parchment-lined roasting pan.
- ❖ Bake for about 15 minutes, rotating the pan once or twice to promote even cooking. Let it cool completely and place in your salad bowl.
- ❖ Toss the asparagus with the vegetables, olive oil, vinegar, mustard and herbs. Salt and pepper to taste.
- ❖ Toss to combine and top with avocado and pine nuts. Enjoy

100) SPECIAL GREEN BEAN CREAM SALAD WITH PINE NUTS

Preparation Time: 10 minutes + chilling time | | **Servings: 5**

Ingredients:

- ✓ 1 ½ pounds green beans, trimmed
- ✓ 2 medium tomatoes, diced
- ✓ 2 bell peppers, seeded and diced
- ✓ 4 tbsp shallots, chopped
- ✓ 1/2 cup pine nuts, roughly chopped
- ✓ 1/2 cup vegan mayonnaise
- ✓ 1 tbsp deli mustard
- ✓ 2 tbsp fresh basil, chopped
- ✓ 2 tbsp fresh parsley, chopped
- ✓ 1/2 tsp red pepper flakes, crushed
- ✓ Sea salt and freshly ground black pepper, to taste

Directions:

- ❖ Boil the green beans in a large saucepan of salted water until they are just tender or about 2 minutes.
- ❖ Drain and let the beans cool completely; then, transfer them to a salad bowl. Toss the beans with the remaining ingredients.
- ❖ Taste and adjust the seasonings. Enjoy

101) EASY KALE CANNELLINI BEAN SOUP

Preparation Time: 25 minutes | | **Servings: 5**

Ingredients:

- ✓ 1 tbsp olive oil
- ✓ 1/2 tsp ginger, minced
- ✓ 1/2 tsp cumin seeds
- ✓ 1 red onion, chopped
- ✓ 1 carrot, trimmed and chopped
- ✓ 1 parsnip, trimmed and chopped
- ✓ 2 garlic cloves, minced
- ✓ 5 cups vegetable broth
- ✓ 12 ounces Cannellini beans, drained
- ✓ 2 cups kale, torn into pieces
- ✓ Sea salt and ground black pepper, to taste

Directions:

- ❖ In a heavy-bottomed pot, heat the olive over medium-high heat. Now, sauté the ginger and cumin for 1 minute or so.
- ❖ Now, add in the onion, carrot and parsnip; continue sautéing an additional 3 minutes or until the vegetables are just tender.
- ❖ Add in the garlic and continue to sauté for 1 minute or until aromatic.
- ❖ Then, pour in the vegetable broth and bring to a boil. Immediately reduce the heat to a simmer and let it cook for 10 minutes.
- ❖ Fold in the Cannellini beans and kale; continue to simmer until the kale wilts and everything is thoroughly heated. Season with salt and pepper to taste.
- ❖ Ladle into individual bowls and serve hot. Enjoy

102) DELICIOUS MUSHROOM SOUP WITH HEARTY CREAM

Preparation Time: 15 minutes | | **Servings: 5**

Ingredients:

- ✓ 2 tbsp soy butter
- ✓ 1 large shallot, chopped
- ✓ 20 ounces Cremini mushrooms, sliced
- ✓ 2 cloves garlic, minced
- ✓ 4 tbsp flaxseed meal
- ✓ 5 cups vegetable broth
- ✓ 1 1/3 cups full-fat coconut milk
- ✓ 1 bay leaf
- ✓ Sea salt and ground black pepper, to taste

Directions:

- ❖ In a stockpot, melt the vegan butter over medium-high heat. Once hot, cook the shallot for about 3 minutes until tender and fragrant.
- ❖ Add in the mushrooms and garlic and continue cooking until the mushrooms have softened. Add in the flaxseed meal and continue to cook for 1 minute or so.
- ❖ Add in the remaining ingredients. Let it simmer, covered and continue to cook for 5 to 6 minutes more until your soup has thickened slightly.
- ❖ Enjoy

103) ITALIAN-STYLE AUTHENTIC PANZANELLA SALAD

Preparation Time: 35 minutes | **Servings: 3**

Ingredients:

- ✓ 3 cups artisan bread, broken into 1-inch cubes
- ✓ 3/4-pound asparagus, trimmed and cut into bite-sized pieces
- ✓ 4 tbsp extra-virgin olive oil
- ✓ 1 red onion, chopped
- ✓ 2 tbsp fresh lime juice
- ✓ 1 tsp deli mustard
- ✓ 2 medium heirloom tomatoes, diced
- ✓ 2 cups arugula
- ✓ 2 cups baby spinach
- ✓ 2 Italian peppers, seeded and sliced
- ✓ Sea salt and ground black pepper, to taste

Directions:

- ❖ Arrange the bread cubes on a parchment-lined baking sheet. Bake in the preheated oven at 310 degrees F for about 20 minutes, rotating the baking sheet twice during the baking time; reserve.
- ❖ Turn the oven to 420 degrees F and toss the asparagus with 1 tbsp of olive oil. Roast the asparagus for about 15 minutes or until crisp-tender.
- ❖ Toss the remaining ingredients in a salad bowl; top with the roasted asparagus and toasted bread.
- ❖ Enjoy

104) ASIAN BLACK BEAN QUINOA SALAD

Preparation Time: 15 minutes + chilling time | **Servings: 4**

Ingredients:

- ✓ 2 cups water
- ✓ 1 cup quinoa, rinsed
- ✓ 16 ounces canned black beans, drained
- ✓ 2 Roma tomatoes, sliced
- ✓ 1 red onion, thinly sliced
- ✓ 1 cucumber, seeded and chopped
- ✓ 2 cloves garlic, pressed or minced
- ✓ 2 Italian peppers, seeded and sliced
- ✓ 2 tbsp fresh parsley, chopped
- ✓ 2 tbsp fresh cilantro, chopped
- ✓ 1/4 cup olive oil
- ✓ 1 lemon, freshly squeezed
- ✓ 1 tbsp apple cider vinegar
- ✓ 1/2 tsp dried dill weed
- ✓ 1/2 tsp dried oregano
- ✓ Sea salt and ground black pepper, to taste

Directions:

- ❖ Place the water and quinoa in a saucepan and bring it to a rolling boil. Immediately turn the heat to a simmer.
- ❖ Let it simmer for about 13 minutes until the quinoa has absorbed all of the water; fluff the quinoa with a fork and let it cool completely. Then, transfer the quinoa to a salad bowl.
- ❖ Add the remaining ingredients to the salad bowl and toss to combine well. Enjoy

105) MOROCCAN POWER BULGUR SALAD WITH HERBS

Preparation Time: 20 minutes + chilling time | **Servings: 4**

Ingredients:

- ✓ 2 cups water
- ✓ 1 cup bulgur
- ✓ 12 ounces canned chickpeas, drained
- ✓ 1 Persian cucumber, thinly sliced
- ✓ 2 bell peppers, seeded and thinly sliced
- ✓ 1 jalapeno pepper, seeded and thinly sliced
- ✓ 2 Roma tomatoes, sliced
- ✓ 1 onion, thinly sliced
- ✓ 2 tbsp fresh basil, chopped
- ✓ 2 tbsp fresh parsley, chopped
- ✓ 2 tbsp fresh mint, chopped
- ✓ 2 tbsp fresh chives, chopped
- ✓ 4 tbsp olive oil
- ✓ 1 tbsp balsamic vinegar
- ✓ 1 tbsp lemon juice
- ✓ 1 tsp fresh garlic, pressed
- ✓ Sea salt and freshly ground black pepper, to taste
- ✓ 2 tbsp nutritional yeast
- ✓ 1/2 cup Kalamata olives, sliced

Directions:

- ❖ In a saucepan, bring the water and bulgur to a boil. Immediately turn the heat to a simmer and let it cook for about 20 minutes or until the bulgur is tender and water is almost absorbed. Fluff with a fork and spread on a large tray to let cool.
- ❖ Place the bulgur in a salad bowl followed by the chickpeas, cucumber, peppers, tomatoes, onion, basil, parsley, mint and chives.
- ❖ In a small mixing dish, whisk the olive oil, balsamic vinegar, lemon juice, garlic, salt and black pepper. Dress the salad and toss to combine.
- ❖ Sprinkle nutritional yeast over the top, garnish with olives and serve at room temperature. Enjoy

106) AUTHENTIC ROASTED PEPPER SALAD

Preparation Time: 15 minutes + chilling time		Servings: 3

Ingredients:

- 6 bell peppers
- 3 tbsp extra-virgin olive oil
- 3 tsp red wine vinegar
- 3 garlic cloves, finely chopped
- 2 tbsp fresh parsley, chopped
- Sea salt and freshly cracked black pepper, to taste
- 1/2 tsp red pepper flakes
- 6 tbsp pine nuts, roughly chopped

Directions:

- Broil the peppers on a parchment-lined baking sheet for about 10 minutes, rotating the pan halfway through the cooking time, until they are charred on all sides.
- Then, cover the peppers with a plastic wrap to steam. Discard the skin, seeds and cores.
- Slice the peppers into strips and toss them with the remaining ingredients. Place in your refrigerator until ready to serve. Enjoy

107) AUTUMN HEARTY QUINOA SOUP

Preparation Time: 25 minutes		Servings: 4

Ingredients:

- 2 tbsp olive oil
- 1 onion, chopped
- 2 carrots, peeled and chopped
- 1 parsnip, chopped
- 1 celery stalk, chopped
- 1 cup yellow squash, chopped
- 4 garlic cloves, pressed or minced
- 4 cups roasted vegetable broth
- 2 medium tomatoes, crushed
- 1 cup quinoa
- Sea salt and ground black pepper, to taste
- 1 bay laurel
- 2 cup Swiss chard, tough ribs removed and torn into pieces
- 2 tbsp Italian parsley, chopped

Directions:

- In a heavy-bottomed pot, heat the olive over medium-high heat. Now, sauté the onion, carrot, parsnip, celery and yellow squash for about 3 minutes or until the vegetables are just tender.
- Add in the garlic and continue to sauté for 1 minute or until aromatic.
- Then, stir in the vegetable broth, tomatoes, quinoa, salt, pepper and bay laurel; bring to a boil. Immediately reduce the heat to a simmer and let it cook for 13 minutes.
- Fold in the Swiss chard; continue to simmer until the chard wilts.
- Ladle into individual bowls and serve garnished with the fresh parsley. Enjoy

108) SPECIAL GREEN LENTIL SALAD

Preparation Time: 20 minutes + chilling time		Servings: 5

Ingredients:

- 1 ½ cups green lentils, rinsed
- 2 cups arugula
- 2 cups Romaine lettuce, torn into pieces
- 1 cup baby spinach
- 1/4 cup fresh basil, chopped
- 1/2 cup shallots, chopped
- 2 garlic cloves, finely chopped
- 1/4 cup oil-packed sun-dried tomatoes, rinsed and chopped
- 5 tbsp extra-virgin olive oil
- 3 tbsp fresh lemon juice
- Sea salt and ground black pepper, to taste

Directions:

- In a large-sized saucepan, bring 4 ½ cups of the water and red lentils to a boil.
- Immediately turn the heat to a simmer and continue to cook your lentils for a further 15 to 17 minutes or until they've softened but not mushy. Drain and let it cool completely.
- Transfer the lentils to a salad bowl; toss the lentils with the remaining ingredients until well combined.
- Serve chilled or at room temperature. Enjoy

47

109) EASY CHICKPEA, ACORN SQUASH, AND COUSCOUS SOUP

Preparation Time: 20 minutes		**Servings:** 4

Ingredients:

- ✓ 2 tbsp olive oil
- ✓ 1 shallot, chopped
- ✓ 1 carrot, trimmed and chopped
- ✓ 2 cups acorn squash, chopped
- ✓ 1 stalk celery, chopped
- ✓ 1 tsp garlic, finely chopped
- ✓ 1 tsp dried rosemary, chopped
- ✓ 1 tsp dried thyme, chopped

- ✓ 2 cups cream of onion soup
- ✓ 2 cups water
- ✓ 1 cup dry couscous
- ✓ Sea salt and ground black pepper, to taste
- ✓ 1/2 tsp red pepper flakes
- ✓ 6 ounces canned chickpeas, drained
- ✓ 2 tbsp fresh lemon juice

Directions:

- ❖ In a heavy-bottomed pot, heat the olive over medium-high heat. Now, sauté the shallot, carrot, acorn squash and celery for about 3 minutes or until the vegetables are just tender.
- ❖ Add in the garlic, rosemary and thyme and continue to sauté for 1 minute or until aromatic.
- ❖ Then, stir in the soup, water, couscous, salt, black pepper and red pepper flakes; bring to a boil. Immediately reduce the heat to a simmer and let it cook for 12 minutes.
- ❖ Fold in the canned chickpeas; continue to simmer until heated through or about 5 minutes more.
- ❖ Ladle into individual bowls and drizzle with the lemon juice over the top. Enjoy

110) SPECIAL PUMPKIN CAYENNE SOUP

Preparation Time: 55 minutes		**Servings:** 6

Ingredients:

- ✓ 1 (2-pound) pumpkin, sliced
- ✓ 3 tbsp olive oil
- ✓ 1 tsp salt
- ✓ 2 red bell peppers
- ✓ 1 onion, halved
- ✓ 1 head garlic

- ✓ 6 cups water
- ✓ Zest and juice of 1 lime
- ✓ ¼ tsp cayenne pepper
- ✓ ½ tsp ground coriander
- ✓ ½ tsp ground cumin
- ✓ Toasted pumpkin seeds

Directions:

- ❖ Preheat oven to 350 F.
- ❖ Brush the pumpkin slices with oil and sprinkle with salt. Arrange the slices skin-side-down and on a greased baking dish and bake for 20 minutes. Brush the onion with oil. Cut the top of the garlic head and brush with oil.
- ❖ When the pumpkin is ready, add in bell peppers, onion, and garlic, and bake for another 10 minutes. Allow cooling.
- ❖ Take out the flesh from the pumpkin skin and transfer to a food processor. Cut the pepper roughly, peel and cut the onion, and remove the cloves from the garlic head. Transfer to the food processor and pour in the water, lime zest, and lime juice.
- ❖ Blend the soup until smooth. If it's very thick, add a bit of water to reach your desired consistency. Sprinkle with salt, cayenne, coriander, and cumin. Serve

111) EASY ZUCCHINI CREAM SOUP WITH WALNUTS

Preparation Time: 45 minutes		**Servings:** 4

Ingredients:

- ✓ 3 zucchinis, chopped
- ✓ 2 tsp olive oil
- ✓ Sea salt and black pepper to taste
- ✓ 1 onion, diced
- ✓ 4 cups vegetable stock

- ✓ 3 tsp ground sage
- ✓ 3 tbsp nutritional yeast
- ✓ 1 cup non-dairy milk
- ✓ ¼ cup toasted walnuts

Directions:

- ❖ Heat the oil in a skillet and place zucchini, onion, salt, and pepper; cook for 5 minutes. Pour in vegetable stock and bring to a boil. Lower the heat and simmer for 15 minutes. Stir in sage, nutritional yeast, and milk. Purée the soup with a blender until smooth. Serve garnished with toasted walnuts and pepper

112)   TRADITIONAL RAMEN SOUP

Preparation Time: 25 minutes		Servings: 4

Ingredients:

- ✓ 7 oz Japanese buckwheat noodles
- ✓ 4 tbsp sesame paste
- ✓ 1 cup canned pinto beans, drained
- ✓ 2 tbsp fresh cilantro, chopped
- ✓ 2 scallions, thinly sliced

Directions:

- ❖ In boiling salted water, add in the noodles and cook for 5 minutes over low heat. Remove a cup of the noodle water to a bowl and add in the sesame paste; stir until it has dissolved. Pour the sesame mix in the pot with the noodles, add in pinto beans, and stir until everything is hot. Serve topped with cilantro and scallions in individual bowls

113)   MEXICAN BLACK-EYED PEA SOUP

Preparation Time: 45 minutes		Servings: 6

Ingredients:

- ✓ 2 carrots, chopped
- ✓ 1 onion, chopped
- ✓ 2 cups canned dried black-eyed peas
- ✓ 1 tbsp soy sauce
- ✓ 3 tsp dried thyme
- ✓ 1 tsp onion powder
- ✓ ½ tsp garlic powder
- ✓ Salt and black pepper to taste
- ✓ ¼ cup chopped pitted black olives

Directions:

- ❖ Place carrots, onion, black-eyed peas, 3 cups water, soy sauce, thyme, onion powder, garlic powder, and pepper in a pot. Bring to a boil, then reduce the heat to low. Cook for 20 minutes. Allow cooling for a few minutes. Transfer to a food processor and blend until smooth. Stir in black olives. Serve

114)   GREEK LEEKS CAULIFLOWER SOUP

Preparation Time: 25 minutes		Servings: 4

Ingredients:

- ✓ 2 tbsp olive oil
- ✓ 3 leeks, thinly sliced
- ✓ 1 head cauliflower, cut into florets
- ✓ 4 cups vegetable stock
- ✓ Salt and black pepper to taste
- ✓ 3 tbsp chopped fresh chives

Directions:

- ❖ Heat the oil in a pot over medium heat. Place the leeks and sauté for 5 minutes. Add in broccoli, vegetable stock, salt, and pepper and cook for 10 minutes. Blend the soup until purée in a food processor. Top with chives and serve

115)   ITALIAN LENTIL LIME SOUP

Preparation Time: 35 minutes		Servings: 2

Ingredients:

- ✓ 1 tsp olive oil
- ✓ 1 onion, chopped
- ✓ 6 garlic cloves, minced
- ✓ 1 tsp chili powder
- ✓ ½ tsp ground cinnamon
- ✓ Salt to taste
- ✓ 1 cup yellow lentils
- ✓ 1 cup canned crushed tomatoes
- ✓ 2 cups water
- ✓ 1 celery stalk, chopped
- ✓ 2 cups chopped collard greens

Directions:

- ❖ Heat oil in a pot over medium heat. Place onion and garlic and cook for 5 minutes. Stir in chili powder, celery, cinnamon, and salt. Pour in lentils, tomatoes and juices, and water. Bring to a boil, then lower the heat and simmer for 15 minutes. Stir in collard greens. Cook for an additional 5 minutes. Serve

116) ASIAN RICE, SPINACH, AND BEAN SOUP

Preparation Time: 45 minutes		Servings: 6

Ingredients:

- ✓ 6 cups baby spinach
- ✓ 2 tbsp olive oil
- ✓ 1 onion, chopped
- ✓ 2 garlic cloves, minced
- ✓ 1 (15.5-oz) can black-eyed peas
- ✓ 6 cups vegetable broth
- ✓ Salt and black pepper to taste
- ✓ ½ cup brown rice
- ✓ Tabasco sauce, for serving

Directions:

- ❖ Heat oil in a pot over medium heat. Place the onion and garlic and sauté for 3 minutes. Pour in broth and season with salt and pepper. Bring to a boil, then lower the heat and stir in rice. Simmer for 15 minutes. Stir in peas and spinach and cook for another 5 minutes. Serve topped with Tabasco sauce

117) CREAMY POTATO SOUP WITH HERBS

Preparation Time: 40 minutes	Servings: 4

Ingredients:

- ✓ 2 tbsp olive oil
- ✓ 1 onion, chopped
- ✓ 1 celery stalk, chopped
- ✓ 4 large potatoes, peeled and chopped
- ✓ 2 garlic cloves, minced
- ✓ 1 tsp fresh basil, chopped
- ✓ 1 tsp fresh parsley, chopped
- ✓ 1 tsp fresh rosemary, chopped
- ✓ 1 bay laurel
- ✓ 1 tsp ground allspice
- ✓ 4 cups vegetable stock
- ✓ Salt and fresh ground black pepper, to taste
- ✓ 2 tbsp fresh chives chopped

Directions:

- ❖ In a heavy-bottomed pot, heat the olive oil over medium-high heat. Once hot, sauté the onion, celery and potatoes for about 5 minutes, stirring periodically.
- ❖ Add in the garlic, basil, parsley, rosemary, bay laurel and allspice and continue sautéing for 1 minute or until fragrant.
- ❖ Now, add in the vegetable stock, salt and black pepper and bring to a rapid boil. Immediately reduce the heat to a simmer and let it cook for about 30 minutes.
- ❖ Puree the soup using an immersion blender until creamy and uniform.
- ❖ Reheat your soup and serve with fresh chives. Enjoy

118)

119) ASIAN QUINOA AND AVOCADO SALAD

Preparation Time: 15 minutes + chilling time		Servings: 4

Ingredients:

- ✓ 1 cup quinoa, rinsed
- ✓ 1 onion, chopped
- ✓ 1 tomato, diced
- ✓ 2 roasted peppers, cut into strips
- ✓ 2 tbsp parsley, chopped
- ✓ 2 tbsp basil, chopped
- ✓ 1/4 cup extra-virgin olive oil
- ✓ 2 tbsp red wine vinegar
- ✓ 2 tbsp lemon juice
- ✓ 1/4 tsp cayenne pepper
- ✓ Sea salt and freshly ground black pepper, to season
- ✓ 1 avocado, peeled, pitted and sliced
- ✓ 1 tbsp sesame seeds, toasted

Directions:

- ❖ Place the water and quinoa in a saucepan and bring it to a rolling boil. Immediately turn the heat to a simmer.
- ❖ Let it simmer for about 13 minutes until the quinoa has absorbed all of the water; fluff the quinoa with a fork and let it cool completely. Then, transfer the quinoa to a salad bowl.
- ❖ Add the onion, tomato, roasted peppers, parsley and basil to the salad bowl. In another small bowl, whisk the olive oil, vinegar, lemon juice, cayenne pepper, salt and black pepper.
- ❖ Dress your salad and toss to combine well. Top with avocado slices and garnish with toasted sesame seeds.
- ❖ Enjoy

120)   VEGETARIAN TABBOULEH SALAD WITH TOFU

Preparation Time: 20 minutes + chilling time

Servings: 4

Ingredients:

- ✓ 1 cup bulgur wheat
- ✓ 2 San Marzano tomatoes, sliced
- ✓ 1 Persian cucumber, thinly sliced
- ✓ 2 tbsp basil, chopped
- ✓ 2 tbsp parsley, chopped
- ✓ 4 scallions, chopped
- ✓ 2 cups arugula
- ✓ 2 cups baby spinach, torn into pieces
- ✓ 4 tbsp tahini
- ✓ 4 tbsp lemon juice
- ✓ 1 tbsp soy sauce
- ✓ 1 tsp fresh garlic, pressed
- ✓ Sea salt and ground black pepper, to taste
- ✓ 12 ounces smoked tofu, cubed

Directions:

- ❖ In a saucepan, bring 2 cups of water and the bulgur to a boil. Immediately turn the heat to a simmer and let it cook for about 20 minutes or until the bulgur is tender and the water is almost absorbed. Fluff with a fork and spread on a large tray to let cool.
- ❖ Place the bulgur in a salad bowl followed by the tomatoes, cucumber, basil, parsley, scallions, arugula and spinach.
- ❖ In a small mixing dish, whisk the tahini, lemon juice, soy sauce, garlic, salt and black pepper. Dress the salad and toss to combine.
- ❖ Top your salad with the smoked tofu and serve at room temperature. Enjoy

121)   SPECIAL GREEN PASTA SALAD

Preparation Time: 10 minutes + chilling time

Servings: 4

Ingredients:

- ✓ 12 ounces rotini pasta
- ✓ 1 small onion, thinly sliced
- ✓ 1 cup cherry tomatoes, halved
- ✓ 1 bell pepper, chopped
- ✓ 1 jalapeno pepper, chopped
- ✓ 1 tbsp capers, drained
- ✓ 2 cups Iceberg lettuce, torn into pieces
- ✓ 2 tbsp fresh parsley, chopped
- ✓ 2 tbsp fresh cilantro, chopped
- ✓ 2 tbsp fresh basil, chopped
- ✓ 1/4 cup olive oil
- ✓ 2 tbsp apple cider vinegar
- ✓ 1 tsp garlic, pressed
- ✓ Kosher salt and ground black pepper, to taste
- ✓ 2 tbsp nutritional yeast
- ✓ 2 tbsp pine nuts, toasted and chopped

Directions:

- ❖ Cook the pasta according to the package directions. Drain and rinse the pasta. Let it cool completely and then, transfer it to a salad bowl.
- ❖ Then, add in the onion, tomatoes, peppers, capers, lettuce, parsley, cilantro and basil to the salad bowl.
- ❖ Whisk the olive oil, vinegar, garlic, salt, black pepper and nutritional yeast. Dress your salad and top with toasted pine nuts. Enjoy

Chapter 3. DINNER

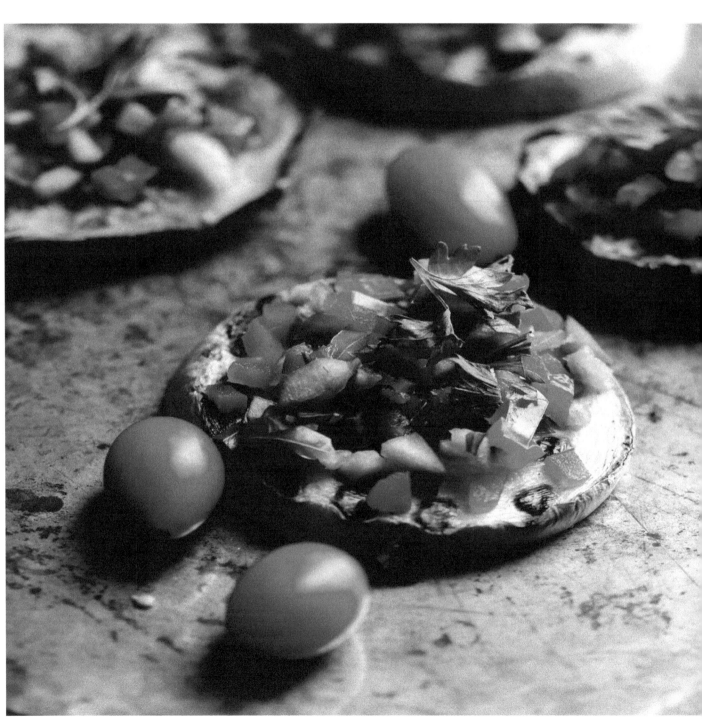

122) ITALIAN MUSHROOM CURRY PIE

Preparation Time: 70 minutes | | **Servings:** 6

Ingredients:

- Piecrust:
- 1 tbsp flax seed powder + 3 tbsp water
- ¾ cup coconut flour
- 4 tbsp chia seeds
- 4 tbsp almond flour
- 1 tbsp psyllium husk powder
- 1 tsp baking powder
- 1 pinch of salt
- 3 tbsp olive oil
- 4 tbsp water

- Filling:
- 1 cup chopped shiitake mushrooms
- 1 cup tofu mayonnaise
- 3 tbsp flax seed powder + 9 tbsp water
- ½ red bell pepper, finely chopped
- 1 tsp turmeric
- ½ tsp paprika
- ½ tsp garlic powder
- ½ cup cashew cream cheese
- 1 ¼ cups grated plant-based Parmesan

Directions:

In two separate bowls, mix the different portions of flax seed powder with the respective quantity of water and set aside to absorb for 5 minutes.

Preheat oven to 350 F. When the vegan "flax egg" is ready, pour the smaller quantity into a food processor, add in the pie crust ingredients and blend until a ball forms out of the dough. Line a springform pan with parchment paper and grease with cooking spray. Spread the dough on the bottom of the pan and bake for 15 minutes. In a bowl, add the remaining flax egg and all the filling ingredients, combine the mixture, and fill the piecrust. Bake for 40 minutes. Serve sliced

123) VEGETARIAN TOFU AND SPINACH LASAGNA WITH RED SAUCE

Preparation Time: 65 minutes | | **Servings:** 4

Ingredients:

- 2 tbsp plant butter
- 1 white onion, chopped
- 1 garlic clove, minced
- 2 ½ cups crumbled tofu
- 3 tbsp tomato paste
- ½ tbsp dried oregano
- Salt and black pepper to taste
- 1 cup baby spinach

- 8 tbsp flax seed powder
- 1 ½ cup cashew cream cheese
- 5 tbsp psyllium husk powder
- 2 cups coconut cream
- 5 oz grated plant-based mozzarella
- 2 oz grated plant-based Parmesan
- ½ cup fresh parsley, finely chopped

Directions:

Melt plant butter in a medium pot and sauté onion and garlic until fragrant and soft, about 3 minutes. Stir in tofu and cook until brown. Mix tomato paste, oregano, salt, and black pepper. Pour ½ cup of water into the pot, stir, and simmer the ingredients until most of the liquid has evaporated.

Preheat oven to 300 F. Mix flax seed powder with 1 ½ cups water in a bowl to make vegan "flax egg." Allow sitting to thicken for 5 minutes. Combine vegan "flax egg" with cashew cream cheese and salt. Add psyllium husk powder a bit at a time while whisking and allow the mixture to sit for a few minutes. Line a baking sheet with parchment paper and spread the mixture in. Cover with another parchment paper and flatten the dough into the sheet. Bake for 10-12 minutes. Slice the pasta into sheets.

In a bowl, combine coconut cream and two-thirds of the plant-based mozzarella cheese. Fetch out 2 tbsp of the mixture and reserve. Mix in plant-based Parmesan cheese, salt, pepper, and parsley. Set aside. Grease a baking dish with cooking spray, layer a single line of pasta, spread with some tomato sauce, 1/3 of the spinach, and ¼ of the coconut cream mixture. Repeat layering the ingredients twice in the same manner, making sure to top the final layer with the coconut cream mixture and the reserved cream cheese. Bake for 30 minutes at 400 F. Slice and serve with salad

53

124) INDIAN CURRIED TOFU WITH BUTTERY CABBAGE

Preparation Time: 55 minutes		Servings: 4

Ingredients:

- ✓ 2 cups tofu, cubed
- ✓ 1 tbsp + 3 ½ tbsp coconut oil
- ✓ ½ cup grated coconut
- ✓ 1 tsp yellow curry powder
- ✓ ½ tsp onion powder
- ✓ 2 cups Napa cabbage, grated
- ✓ 4 oz plant butter
- ✓ Salt and black pepper to taste
- ✓ Lemon wedges for serving

Directions:

Drizzle 1 tbsp of coconut oil on the tofu. In a bowl, mix the shredded coconut, yellow curry powder, salt, and onion powder. Toss the tofu cubes in the spice mixture. Heat the remaining coconut oil in a non-stick skillet and fry the coated tofu until golden brown on all sides. Transfer to a plate.

In another skillet, melt half of the plant butter, add, and sauté the cabbage until slightly caramelized. Then, season with salt and black pepper. Dish the cabbage into serving plates with the tofu and lemon wedges. Melt the remaining plant butter in the skillet and drizzle over the cabbage and tofu. Serve

125) SIMPLE AVOCADO COCONUT PIE

Preparation Time: 80 minutes		Servings: 4

Ingredients:

- ✓ Piecrust:
- ✓ 1 tbsp flax seed powder + 3 tbsp water
- ✓ 1 cup coconut flour
- ✓ 4 tbsp chia seeds
- ✓ 1 tbsp psyllium husk powder
- ✓ 1 tsp baking soda
- ✓ 1 pinch salt
- ✓ 3 tbsp coconut oil
- ✓ 4 tbsp water
- ✓ Filling:
- ✓ 2 ripe avocados, chopped
- ✓ 1 cup tofu mayonnaise
- ✓ 3 tbsp flax seed powder + 9 tbsp water
- ✓ 2 tbsp fresh parsley, chopped
- ✓ 1 jalapeno, finely chopped
- ✓ ½ tsp onion powder
- ✓ ¼ tsp salt
- ✓ ½ cup cream cheese
- ✓ 1 ¼ cups grated plant-based Parmesan

Directions:

In 2 separate bowls, mix the different portions of flax seed powder with the respective quantity of water. Allow absorbing for 5 minutes.

Preheat oven to 350 F. In a food processor, add the piecrust ingredients and the smaller portion of the vegan "flax egg." Blend until the resulting dough forms into a ball. Line a springform pan with parchment paper and spread the dough in the pan. Bake for 10-15 minutes.

Put the avocado in a bowl and add the tofu mayonnaise, remaining vegan "flax egg," parsley, jalapeno, onion powder, salt, cream cheese, and plant-based Parmesan. Combine well. Remove the piecrust when ready and fill with the creamy mixture. Bake for 35 minutes. Cool before slicing and serving

126) EASY GREEN AVOCADO CARBONARA

Preparation Time: 30 minutes		Servings: 4

Ingredients:

- ✓ 8 tbsp flax seed powder
- ✓ 1 ½ cups cashew cream cheese
- ✓ 5 ½ tbsp psyllium husk powder
- ✓ 1 avocado, chopped
- ✓ 1 ¾ cups coconut cream
- ✓ Juice of ½ lemon
- ✓ 1 tsp onion powder
- ✓ ½ tsp garlic powder
- ✓ ¼ cup olive oil
- ✓ Salt and black pepper to taste
- ✓ ½ cup grated plant-based Parmesan
- ✓ 4 tbsp toasted pecans

Directions:

Preheat oven to 300 F.

In a medium bowl, mix the flax seed powder with 1 ½ cups water and allow sitting to thicken for 5 minutes. Add the cashew cream cheese, salt, and psyllium husk powder. Whisk until smooth batter forms. Line a baking sheet with parchment paper, pour in the batter, and cover with another parchment paper. Use a rolling pin to flatten the dough into the sheet. Bake for 10-12 minutes. Remove, take off the parchment papers and use a sharp knife to slice the pasta into thin strips lengthwise. Cut each piece into halves, pour into a bowl, and set aside.

In a blender, combine avocado, coconut cream, lemon juice, onion powder, and garlic powder; puree until smooth. Pour the olive oil over the pasta and stir to coat properly. Pour the avocado sauce on top and mix. Season with salt and black pepper. Divide the pasta into serving plates, garnish with Parmesan cheese and pecans, and serve immediately

127) QUICK MUSHROOM AND GREEN BEAN BIRYANI

Preparation Time: 50 minutes		Servings: 4

Ingredients:

- 1 cup brown rice
- 3 tbsp plant butter
- 3 medium white onions, chopped
- 6 garlic cloves, minced
- 1 tsp ginger puree
- 1 tbsp turmeric powder + for dusting
- ¼ tsp cinnamon powder
- 2 tsp garam masala
- ½ tsp cardamom powder
- ½ tsp cayenne powder
- ½ tsp cumin powder
- 1 tsp smoked paprika
- 3 large tomatoes, diced
- 2 green chilies, minced
- 1 tbsp tomato puree
- 1 cup chopped cremini mushrooms
- 1 cup chopped mustard greens
- 1 cup plant-based yogurt

Directions:

Melt the butter in a large pot and sauté the onions until softened, 3 minutes. Mix in the garlic, ginger, turmeric, cardamom powder, garam masala, cardamom powder, cayenne pepper, cumin powder, paprika, and salt. Stir-fry for 1-2 minutes.

Stir in the tomatoes, green chili, tomato puree, and mushrooms. Once boiling, mix in the rice and cover with water. Cover the pot and cook over medium heat until the liquid absorbs and the rice is tender, 15-20 minutes. Open the lid and fluff in the mustard greens and half of the parsley. Dish the food, top with the coconut yogurt, garnish with the remaining parsley, and serve warm

128) TASTY BAKED CHEESY SPAGHETTI SQUASH

Preparation Time: 40 minutes		Servings: 4

Ingredients:

- 2 lb spaghetti squash
- 1 tbsp coconut oil
- Salt and black pepper to taste
- 2 tbsp melted plant butter
- ½ tbsp garlic powder
- 1/5 tsp chili powder
- 1 cup coconut cream
- 2 oz cashew cream cheese
- 1 cup plant-based mozzarella
- 2 oz grated plant-based Parmesan
- 2 tbsp fresh cilantro, chopped
- Olive oil for drizzling

Directions:

Preheat oven to 350 F.

Cut the squash in halves lengthwise and spoon out the seeds and fiber. Place on a baking dish, brush with coconut oil, and season with salt and pepper. Bake for 30 minutes. Remove and use two forks to shred the flesh into strands.

Empty the spaghetti strands into a bowl and mix with plant butter, garlic and chili powders, coconut cream, cream cheese, half of the plant-based mozzarella and plant-based Parmesan cheeses. Spoon the mixture into the squash cups and sprinkle with the remaining mozzarella cheese. Bake further for 5 minutes. Sprinkle with cilantro and drizzle with some oil. Serve

129) KALE AND MUSHROOM PIEROGIS

Preparation Time: 45 minutes		Servings: 4

Ingredients:

- Stuffing:
- 2 tbsp plant butter
- 2 garlic cloves, finely chopped
- 1 small red onion, finely chopped
- 3 oz baby Bella mushrooms, sliced
- 2 oz fresh kale
- ½ tsp salt
- ¼ tsp freshly ground black pepper
- ½ cup dairy-free cream cheese
- 2 oz plant-based Parmesan, grated
- Pierogi:
- 1 tbsp flax seed powder
- ½ cup almond flour
- 4 tbsp coconut flour
- ½ tsp salt
- 1 tsp baking powder
- 1 ½ cups grated plant-based Parmesan
- 5 tbsp plant butter
- Olive oil for brushing

Directions:

Put the plant butter in a skillet and melt over medium heat, then add and sauté the garlic, red onion, mushrooms, and kale until the mushrooms brown. Season the mixture with salt and black pepper and reduce the heat to low. Stir in the cream cheese and plant-based Parmesan cheese and simmer for 1 minute. Turn the heat off and set the filling aside to cool.

Make the pierogis: In a small bowl, mix the flax seed powder with 3 tbsp water and allow sitting for 5 minutes. In a bowl, combine almond flour, coconut flour, salt, and baking powder. Put a small pan over low heat, add, and melt the plant-based Parmesan cheese and plant butter while stirring continuously until smooth batter forms. Turn the heat off.

Pour the vegan "flax egg" into the cream mixture, continue stirring while adding the flour mixture until a firm dough forms. Mold the dough into four balls, place on a chopping board, and use a rolling pin to flatten each into ½ inch thin round pieces. Spread a generous amount of stuffing on one-half of each dough, then fold over the filling, and seal the dough with your fingers. Brush with olive oil, place on a baking sheet, and bake for 20 minutes at 380 F. Serve with salad

130) SPECIAL VEGAN MUSHROOM PIZZA

Preparation Time: 35 minutes | | **Servings:** 4

Ingredients:

- ✓ 2 tsp plant butter
- ✓ 1 cup chopped button mushrooms
- ✓ ½ cup sliced mixed bell peppers
- ✓ Salt and black pepper to taste
- ✓ 1 pizza crust
- ✓ 1 cup tomato sauce
- ✓ 1 cup plant-based Parmesan cheese
- ✓ 5-6 basil leaves

Directions:

Melt plant butter in a skillet and sauté mushrooms and bell peppers for 10 minutes until softened. Season with salt and black pepper. Put the pizza crust on a pizza pan, spread the tomato sauce all over, and scatter vegetables evenly on top. Sprinkle with plant-based Parmesan cheese. Bake for 20 minutes until the cheese has melted. Garnish with basil and serve

---

131) ONLY GRILLED ZUCCHINI WITH SPINACH AVOCADO PESTO

Preparation Time: 20 minutes | | **Servings:** 4

Ingredients:

- ✓ 3 oz spinach, chopped
- ✓ 1 ripe avocado, chopped
- ✓ Juice of 1 lemon
- ✓ 1 garlic clove, minced
- ✓ 2 oz pecans
- ✓ Salt and black pepper to taste
- ✓ ¾ cup olive oil
- ✓ 2 zucchini, sliced
- ✓ 1 tbsp fresh lemon juice
- ✓ 2 tbsp melted plant butter
- ✓ 1 ½ lb tempeh slices

Directions:

Place the spinach in a food processor along with the avocado, lemon juice, garlic, and pecans. Blend until smooth and then season with salt and black pepper. Add the olive oil and process a little more. Pour the pesto into a bowl and set aside.

Place zucchini in a bowl. Season with the remaining lemon juice, salt, black pepper, and the plant butter. Also, season the tempeh with salt and black pepper, and brush with olive oil. Preheat a grill pan and cook both the tempeh and zucchini slices until browned on both sides. Plate the tempeh and zucchini, spoon some pesto to the side, and serve immediately

132) BEST EGGPLANT FRIES WITH CHILI AIOLI AND BEET SALAD

Preparation Time: 35 minutes

Servings: 4

Ingredients:

- ✓ Eggplant Fries:
- ✓ 2 tbsp flax seed powder
- ✓ 2 eggplants, sliced
- ✓ 2 cups almond flour
- ✓ Salt and black pepper to taste
- ✓ 2 tbsp olive oil
- ✓ Beet salad:
- ✓ 3½ oz beets, peeled and thinly cut
- ✓ 3½ oz red cabbage, grated
- ✓ 2 tbsp fresh cilantro
- ✓ 2 tbsp olive oil
- ✓ 1 tbsp freshly squeezed lime juice
- ✓ Salt and black pepper to taste
- ✓ Spicy Aioli:
- ✓ 1 tbsp flax seed powder
- ✓ 2 garlic cloves, minced
- ✓ ¾ cup light olive oil
- ✓ ½ tsp red chili flakes
- ✓ 1 tbsp freshly squeezed lemon juice
- ✓ 3 tbsp dairy-free yogurt

Directions:

Preheat oven to 400 F. In a bowl, combine the flax seed powder with 6 tbsp water and allow sitting to thicken for 5 minutes. In a deep plate, mix almond flour, salt, and black pepper. Dip the eggplant slices into the vegan "flax egg," then in the almond flour, and then in the vegan "flax egg," and finally in the flour mixture. Place the eggplants on a greased baking sheet and drizzle with olive oil. Bake until the fries are crispy and brown, about 15 minutes.

For the aioli, mix the flax seed powder with 3 tbsp water in a bowl and set aside to thicken for 5 minutes. Whisk in garlic while pouring in the olive oil gradually. Stir in red chili flakes, salt, black pepper, lemon juice, and dairy-free yogurt. Adjust the taste with salt, garlic, or yogurt as desired.

For the beet salad, in a salad bowl, combine the beets, red cabbage, cilantro, olive oil, lime juice, salt, and black pepper. Use two spoons to toss the ingredients until properly combined. Serve the eggplant fries with the chili aioli and beet salad

133)

133) BEST TOFU SKEWERS WITH SALSA VERDE AND SQUASH MASH

Preparation Time: 20 minutes

Servings: 4

Ingredients:

- ✓ 7 tbsp fresh cilantro, finely chopped
- ✓ 4 tbsp fresh basil, finely chopped
- ✓ 2 garlic cloves
- ✓ Juice of ½ lemon
- ✓ 4 tbsp capers
- ✓ ⅔ cup olive oil
- ✓ 1 lb extra firm tofu, cubed
- ✓ ½ tbsp sugar-free BBQ sauce
- ✓ 1 tbsp melted plant butter
- ✓ 3 cups butternut squash, cubed
- ✓ ½ cup cold plant butter
- ✓ 2 oz grated plant-based Parmesan

Directions:

In a blender, add cilantro, basil, garlic, lemon juice, capers, olive oil, salt, and pepper. Process until smooth; set aside. Thread the tofu cubes on wooden skewers. Season with salt and brush with BBQ sauce. Melt plant butter in a grill pan and fry the tofu until browned. Remove to a plate. Pour the squash into a pot, add some lightly salted water, and bring the vegetable to a boil until soft, about 6 minutes. Drain and pour into a bowl. Add the cold plant butter, plant-based Parmesan cheese, salt, and black pepper. Mash the vegetable with an immersion blender until the consistency of mashed potatoes is achieved. Serve the tofu skewers with the mashed cauliflower and salsa verde

134) SPECIAL MUSHROOM LETTUCE WRAPS

Preparation Time: 25 minutes

Servings: 4

Ingredients:

- ✓ 2 tbsp plant butter
- ✓ 4 oz baby Bella mushrooms, sliced
- ✓ 1 ½ lb tofu, crumbled
- ✓ 1 iceberg lettuce, leaves extracted
- ✓ 1 cup grated plant-based cheddar
- ✓ 1 large tomato, sliced

Directions:

Melt the plant butter in a skillet, add in mushrooms and sauté until browned and tender, about 6 minutes. Transfer to a plate. Add the tofu to the skillet and cook until brown, about 10 minutes. Spoon the tofu and mushrooms into the lettuce leaves, sprinkle with the plant-based cheddar cheese, and share the tomato slices on top. Serve the burger immediately

135)   ORIGINAL GARLICKY RICE

Preparation Time: 20 minutes		Servings: 4

Ingredients:

- ✓ 4 tbsp olive oil
- ✓ 4 cloves garlic, chopped

- ✓ 1 ½ cups white rice
- ✓ 2 ½ cups vegetable broth

Directions:

In a saucepan, heat the olive oil over a moderately high flame. Add in the garlic and sauté for about 1 minute or until aromatic.

Add in the rice and broth. Bring to a boil; immediately turn the heat to a gentle simmer.

Cook for about 15 minutes or until all the liquid has absorbed. Fluff the rice with a fork, season with salt and pepper and serve hot

136)   CLASSIC BROWN RICE WITH VEGETABLES AND TOFU

Preparation Time: 45 minutes		Servings: 4

Ingredients:

- ✓ 4 tsp sesame seeds
- ✓ 2 spring garlic stalks, minced
- ✓ 1 cup spring onions, chopped
- ✓ 1 carrot, trimmed and sliced
- ✓ 1 celery rib, sliced
- ✓ 1/4 cup dry white wine

- ✓ 10 ounces tofu, cubed
- ✓ 1 ½ cups long-grain brown rice, rinsed thoroughly
- ✓ 2 tbsp soy sauce
- ✓ 2 tbsp tahini
- ✓ 1 tbsp lemon juice

Directions:

In a wok or large saucepan, heat 2 tsp of the sesame oil over medium-high heat. Now, cook the garlic, onion, carrot and celery for about 3 minutes, stirring periodically to ensure even cooking.

Add the wine to deglaze the pan and push the vegetables to one side of the wok. Add in the remaining sesame oil and fry the tofu for 8 minutes, stirring occasionally.

Bring 2 ½ cups of water to a boil over medium-high heat. Bring to a simmer and cook the rice for about 30 minutes or until it is tender; fluff the rice and stir it with the soy sauce and tahini.

Stir the vegetables and tofu into the hot rice; add a few drizzles of the fresh lemon juice and serve warm. Enjoy

137)   SIMPLE AMARANTH PORRIDGE

Preparation Time: 35 minutes		Servings: 4

Ingredients:

- ✓ 3 cups water
- ✓ 1 cup amaranth
- ✓ 1/2 cup coconut milk

- ✓ 4 tbsp agave syrup
- ✓ A pinch of kosher salt
- ✓ A pinch of grated nutmeg

Directions:

Bring the water to a boil over medium-high heat; add in the amaranth and turn the heat to a simmer.

Let it cook for about 30 minutes, stirring periodically to prevent the amaranth from sticking to the bottom of the pan.

Stir in the remaining ingredients and continue to cook for 1 to 2 minutes more until cooked through. Enjoy

138) CLASSIC COUNTRY CORNBREAD WITH SPINACH

Preparation Time: 50 minutes		Servings: 8

Ingredients:

- ✓ 1 tbsp flaxseed meal
- ✓ 1 cup all-purpose flour
- ✓ 1 cup yellow cornmeal
- ✓ 1/2 tsp baking soda
- ✓ 1/2 tsp baking powder
- ✓ 1 tsp kosher salt
- ✓ 1 tsp brown sugar
- ✓ A pinch of grated nutmeg
- ✓ 1 ¼ cups oat milk, unsweetened
- ✓ 1 tsp white vinegar
- ✓ 1/2 cup olive oil
- ✓ 2 cups spinach, torn into pieces

Directions:

Start by preheating your oven to 420 degrees F. Now, spritz a baking pan with a nonstick cooking spray.

To make the flax eggs, mix flaxseed meal with 3 tbsp of the water. Stir and let it sit for about 15 minutes.

In a mixing bowl, thoroughly combine the flour, cornmeal, baking soda, baking powder, salt, sugar and grated nutmeg.

Gradually add in the flax egg, oat milk, vinegar and olive oil, whisking constantly to avoid lumps. Afterwards, fold in the spinach.

Scrape the batter into the prepared baking pan. Bake your cornbread for about 25 minutes or until a tester inserted in the middle comes out dry and clean.

Let it stand for about 10 minutes before slicing and serving. Enjoy

139) SIMPLE RICE PUDDING WITH CURRANTS

Preparation Time: 45 minutes		Servings: 4

Ingredients:

- ✓ 1 ½ cups water
- ✓ 1 cup white rice
- ✓ 2 ½ cups oat milk, divided
- ✓ 1/2 cup white sugar
- ✓ A pinch of salt
- ✓ A pinch of grated nutmeg
- ✓ 1 tsp ground cinnamon
- ✓ 1/2 tsp vanilla extract
- ✓ 1/2 cup dried currants

Directions:

In a saucepan, bring the water to a boil over medium-high heat. Immediately turn the heat to a simmer, add in the rice and let it cook for about 20 minutes.

Add in the milk, sugar and spices and continue to cook for 20 minutes more, stirring constantly to prevent the rice from sticking to the pan.

Top with dried currants and serve at room temperature. Enjoy

140) EASY MILLET PORRIDGE WITH SULTANAS

Preparation Time: 25 minutes		Servings: 3

Ingredients:

- ✓ 1 cup water
- ✓ 1 cup coconut milk
- ✓ 1 cup millet, rinsed
- ✓ 1/4 tsp grated nutmeg
- ✓ 1/4 tsp ground cinnamon
- ✓ 1 tsp vanilla paste
- ✓ 1/4 tsp kosher salt
- ✓ 2 tbsp agave syrup
- ✓ 4 tbsp sultana raisins

Directions:

Place the water, milk, millet, nutmeg, cinnamon, vanilla and salt in a saucepan; bring to a boil.

Turn the heat to a simmer and let it cook for about 20 minutes; fluff the millet with a fork and spoon into individual bowls.

Serve with agave syrup and sultanas. Enjoy

141)   ENGLISH QUINOA PORRIDGE WITH DRIED FIGS

Preparation Time: 25 minutes

Servings: 3

Ingredients:

- ✓ 1 cup white quinoa, rinsed
- ✓ 2 cups almond milk
- ✓ 4 tbsp brown sugar
- ✓ A pinch of salt
- ✓ 1/4 tsp grated nutmeg
- ✓ 1/2 tsp ground cinnamon
- ✓ 1/2 tsp vanilla extract
- ✓ 1/2 cup dried figs, chopped

Directions:

Place the quinoa, almond milk, sugar, salt, nutmeg, cinnamon and vanilla extract in a saucepan.

Bring it to a boil over medium-high heat. Turn the heat to a simmer and let it cook for about 20 minutes; fluff with a fork.

Divide between three serving bowls and garnish with dried figs. Enjoy

142)   DELICIOUS SWEET AND SPICY BRUSSEL SPROUT STIR-FRY

Preparation Time: 15 minutes

Servings: 4

Ingredients:

- ✓ 4 oz plant butter + more to taste
- ✓ 4 shallots, chopped
- ✓ 1 tbsp apple cider vinegar
- ✓ Salt and black pepper to taste
- ✓ 1 lb Brussels sprouts
- ✓ Hot chili sauce

Directions:

Put the plant butter in a saucepan and melt over medium heat. Pour in the shallots and sauté for 2 minutes, to caramelize and slightly soften. Add the apple cider vinegar, salt, and black pepper. Stir and reduce the heat to cook the shallots further with continuous stirring, about 5 minutes. Transfer to a plate after.

Trim the Brussel sprouts and cut in halves. Leave the small ones as wholes. Pour the Brussel sprouts into the saucepan and stir-fry with more plant butter until softened but al dente. Season with salt and black pepper, stir in the onions and hot chili sauce, and heat for a few seconds. Serve immediately

143)   MEXICAN BLACK BEAN BURGERS WITH BBQ SAUCE

Preparation Time: 20 minutes

Servings: 4

Ingredients:

- ✓ 3 (15 oz) cans black beans, drained
- ✓ 2 tbsp whole-wheat flour
- ✓ 2 tbsp quick-cooking oats
- ✓ ¼ cup chopped fresh basil
- ✓ 2 tbsp pure barbecue sauce
- ✓ 1 garlic clove, minced
- ✓ Salt and black pepper to taste
- ✓ 4 whole-grain hamburger buns, split
- ✓ For topping:
- Red onion slices
- Tomato slices
- Fresh basil leaves
- Additional barbecue sauce

Directions:

In a medium bowl, mash the black beans and mix in the flour, oats, basil, barbecue sauce, garlic salt, and black pepper until well combined. Mold 4 patties out of the mixture and set aside.

Heat a grill pan to medium heat and lightly grease with cooking spray. Cook the bean patties on both sides until light brown and cooked through, 10 minutes. Place the patties between the burger buns and top with the onions, tomatoes, basil, and some barbecue sauce. Serve warm

144)   LOVELY CREAMY BRUSSELS SPROUTS BAKE

Preparation Time: 26 minutes

Servings: 4

Ingredients:

- ✓ 3 tbsp plant butter
- ✓ 1 cup tempeh, cut into 1-inch cubes
- ✓ 1 ½ lb halved Brussels sprouts
- ✓ 5 garlic cloves, minced
- ✓ 1 ¼ cups coconut cream
- ✓ 10 oz grated plant-based mozzarella
- ✓ ¼ cup grated plant-based Parmesan
- ✓ Salt and black pepper to taste

Preheat oven to 400 F.

Melt the plant butter in a large skillet over medium heat and fry the tempeh cubes until browned on both sides, about 6 minutes. Remove onto a plate and set aside. Pour the Brussels sprouts and garlic into the skillet and sauté until fragrant.

Mix in coconut cream and simmer for 4 minutes. Add tempeh cubes and combine well. Pour the sauté into a baking dish, sprinkle with plant-based mozzarella cheese, and plant-based Parmesan cheese. Bake for 10 minutes or until golden brown on top. Serve with tomato salad

145) GENOVESE BASIL PESTO SEITAN PANINI

Preparation Time: 15 minutes+ cooling time

Servings: 4

Ingredients:

- ✓ For the seitan:
- ✓ 2/3 cup basil pesto
- ✓ ½ lemon, juiced
- ✓ 1 garlic clove, minced
- ✓ 1/8 tsp salt
- ✓ 1 cup chopped seitan
- ✓ For the panini:
- ✓ 3 tbsp basil pesto
- ✓ 8 thick slices whole-wheat ciabatta
- ✓ Olive oil for brushing
- ✓ 8 slices plant-based mozzarella
- ✓ 1 yellow bell pepper, chopped
- ✓ ¼ cup grated plant Parmesan cheese

Directions:

In a medium bowl, mix the pesto, lemon juice, garlic, and salt. Add the seitan and coat well with the marinade. Cover with plastic wrap and marinate in the refrigerator for 30 minutes.

Preheat a large skillet over medium heat and remove the seitan from the fridge. Cook the seitan in the skillet until brown and cooked through, 2-3 minutes. Turn the heat off.

Preheat a panini press to medium heat. In a small bowl, mix the pesto in the inner parts of two slices of bread. On the outer parts, apply some olive oil and place a slice with (the olive oil side down) in the press. Lay 2 slices of plant-based mozzarella cheese on the bread, spoon some seitan on top. Sprinkle with some bell pepper and some plant-based Parmesan cheese. Cover with another bread slice.

Close the press and grill the bread for 1 to 2 minutes. Flip the bread, and grill further for 1 minute or until the cheese melts and golden brown on both sides. Serve warm

146) ENGLISH SWEET OATMEAL "GRITS"

Preparation Time: 20 minutes

Servings: 4

Ingredients:

- ✓ 1 ½ cups steel-cut oats, soaked overnight
- ✓ 1 cup almond milk
- ✓ 2 cups water
- ✓ A pinch of grated nutmeg
- ✓ A pinch of ground cloves
- ✓ A pinch of sea salt
- ✓ 4 tbsp almonds, slivered
- ✓ 6 dates, pitted and chopped
- ✓ 6 prunes, chopped

Directions:

In a deep saucepan, bring the steel cut oats, almond milk and water to a boil.

Add in the nutmeg, cloves and salt. Immediately turn the heat to a simmer, cover and continue to cook for about 15 minutes or until they've softened.

Then, spoon the grits into four serving bowls; top them with the almonds, dates and prunes.

Enjoy!

147) SPECIAL FREEKEH BOWL WITH DRIED FIGS

Preparation Time: 35 minutes

Servings: 2

Ingredients:

- ✓ 1/2 cup freekeh, soaked for 30 minutes, drained
- ✓ 1 1/3 cups almond milk
- ✓ 1/4 tsp sea salt
- ✓ 1/4 tsp ground cloves
- ✓ 1/4 tsp ground cinnamon
- ✓ 4 tbsp agave syrup
- ✓ 2 ounces dried figs, chopped

Directions:

Place the freekeh, milk, sea salt, ground cloves and cinnamon in a saucepan. Bring to a boil over medium-high heat.

Immediately turn the heat to a simmer for 30 to 35 minutes, stirring occasionally to promote even cooking.

Stir in the agave syrup and figs. Ladle the porridge into individual bowls and serve. Enjoy

148) EASY CORNMEAL PORRIDGE WITH MAPLE SYRUP

Preparation Time: 20 minutes		Servings: 4

Ingredients:

- ✓ 2 cups water
- ✓ 2 cups almond milk
- ✓ 1 cinnamon stick
- ✓ 1 vanilla bean
- ✓ 1 cup yellow cornmeal
- ✓ 1/2 cup maple syrup

Directions:

In a saucepan, bring the water and almond milk to a boil. Add in the cinnamon stick and vanilla bean.

Gradually add in the cornmeal, stirring continuously; turn the heat to a simmer. Let it simmer for about 15 minutes.

Drizzle the maple syrup over the porridge and serve warm. Enjoy

149) EVERYDAY MEDITERRANEAN-STYLE RICE

Preparation Time: 20 minutes		Servings: 4

Ingredients:

- ✓ 3 tbsp vegan butter, at room temperature
- ✓ 4 tbsp scallions, chopped
- ✓ 2 cloves garlic, minced
- ✓ 1 bay leaf
- ✓ 1 thyme sprig, chopped
- ✓ 1 rosemary sprig, chopped
- ✓ 1 ½ cups white rice
- ✓ 2 cups vegetable broth
- ✓ 1 large tomato, pureed
- ✓ Sea salt and ground black pepper, to taste
- ✓ 2 ounces Kalamata olives, pitted and sliced

Directions:

In a saucepan, melt the vegan butter over a moderately high flame. Cook the scallions for about 2 minutes or until tender.

Add in the garlic, bay leaf, thyme and rosemary and continue to sauté for about 1 minute or until aromatic.

Add in the rice, broth and pureed tomato. Bring to a boil; immediately turn the heat to a gentle simmer.

Cook for about 15 minutes or until all the liquid has absorbed. Fluff the rice with a fork, season with salt and pepper and garnish with olives; serve immediately. Enjoy

150) MOROCCAN BULGUR PANCAKES WITH A TWIST

Preparation Time: 50 minutes		Servings: 4

Ingredients:

- ✓ 1/2 cup bulgur wheat flour
- ✓ 1/2 cup almond flour
- ✓ 1 tsp baking soda
- ✓ 1/2 tsp fine sea salt
- ✓ 1 cup full-fat coconut milk
- ✓ 1/2 tsp ground cinnamon
- ✓ 1/4 tsp ground cloves
- ✓ 4 tbsp coconut oil
- ✓ 1/2 cup maple syrup
- ✓ 1 large-sized banana, sliced

Directions:

In a mixing bowl, thoroughly combine the flour, baking soda, salt, coconut milk, cinnamon and ground cloves; let it stand for 30 minutes to soak well.

Heat a small amount of the coconut oil in a frying pan.

Fry the pancakes until the surface is golden brown. Garnish with maple syrup and banana. Enjoy

151) SIMPLE CHOCOLATE RYE PORRIDGE

Preparation Time: 10 minutes		Servings: 4

Ingredients:

- ✓ 2 cups rye flakes
- ✓ 2 ½ cups almond milk
- ✓ 2 ounces dried prunes, chopped
- ✓ 2 ounces dark chocolate chunks

Directions:

Add the rye flakes and almond milk to a deep saucepan; bring to a boil over medium-high. Turn the heat to a simmer and let it cook for 5 to 6 minutes.

Remove from the heat. Fold in the chopped prunes and chocolate chunks, gently stir to combine.

Ladle into serving bowls and serve warm.

Enjoy

152) CLASSIC AFRICAN MIELIE-MEAL

Preparation Time: 15 minutes		Servings: 4

Ingredients:

- ✓ 3 cups water
- ✓ 1 cup coconut milk
- ✓ 1 cup maize meal
- ✓ 1/3 tsp kosher salt
- ✓ 1/4 tsp grated nutmeg
- ✓ 1/4 tsp ground cloves
- ✓ 4 tbsp maple syrup

Directions:

In a saucepan, bring the water and milk to a boil; then, gradually add in the maize meal and turn the heat to a simmer.

Add in the salt, nutmeg and cloves. Let it cook for 10 minutes.

Add in the maple syrup and gently stir to combine. Enjoy

153) SPECIAL TEFF PORRIDGE WITH DRIED FIGS

Preparation Time: 25 minutes		Servings: 4

Ingredients:

- ✓ 1 cup whole-grain teff
- ✓ 1 cup water
- ✓ 2 cups coconut milk
- ✓ 2 tbsp coconut oil
- ✓ 1/2 tsp ground cardamom
- ✓ 1/4 tsp ground cinnamon
- ✓ 4 tbsp agave syrup
- ✓ 7-8 dried figs, chopped

Directions:

Bring the whole-grain teff, water and coconut milk to a boil.

Turn the heat to a simmer and add in the coconut oil, cardamom and cinnamon.

Let it cook for 20 minutes or until the grain has softened and the porridge has thickened. Stir in the agave syrup and stir to combine well.

Top each serving bowl with chopped figs and serve warm. Enjoy

154) TASTY DECADENT BREAD PUDDING WITH APRICOTS

Preparation Time: 1 hour		Servings: 4

Ingredients:

- ✓ 4 cups day-old ciabatta bread, cubed
- ✓ 4 tbsp coconut oil, melted
- ✓ 2 cups coconut milk
- ✓ 1/2 cup coconut sugar
- ✓ 4 tbsp applesauce
- ✓ 1/4 tsp ground cloves
- ✓ 1/2 tsp ground cinnamon
- ✓ 1 tsp vanilla extract
- ✓ 1/3 cup dried apricots, diced

Directions:

Start by preheating your oven to 360 degrees F. Lightly oil a casserole dish with a nonstick cooking spray.

Place the cubed bread in the prepared casserole dish.

In a mixing bowl, thoroughly combine the coconut oil, milk, coconut sugar, applesauce, ground cloves, ground cinnamon and vanilla. Pour the custard evenly over the bread cubes; fold in the apricots.

Press with a wide spatula and let it soak for about 15 minutes.

Bake in the preheated oven for about 45 minutes or until the top is golden and set. Enjoy

155) TRADITIONAL CHIPOTLE CILANTRO RICE

Preparation Time: 25 minutes		Servings: 4

Ingredients:

- ✓ 4 tbsp olive oil
- ✓ 1 chipotle pepper, seeded and chopped
- ✓ 1 cup jasmine rice
- ✓ 1 ½ cups vegetable broth
- ✓ 1/4 cup fresh cilantro, chopped
- ✓ Sea salt and cayenne pepper, to taste

Directions:

In a saucepan, heat the olive oil over a moderately high flame. Add in the pepper and rice and cook for about 3 minutes or until aromatic.

Pour the vegetable broth into the saucepan and bring to a boil; immediately turn the heat to a gentle simmer.

Cook for about 18 minutes or until all the liquid has absorbed. Fluff the rice with a fork, add in the cilantro, salt and cayenne pepper; stir to combine well. Enjoy

156) ENGLISH OAT PORRIDGE WITH ALMONDS

Preparation Time: 20 minutes		Servings: 2

Ingredients:

- ✓ 1 cup water
- ✓ 2 cups almond milk, divided
- ✓ 1 cup rolled oats
- ✓ 2 tbsp coconut sugar
- ✓ 1/2 vanilla essence
- ✓ 1/4 tsp cardamom
- ✓ 1/2 cup almonds, chopped
- ✓ 1 banana, sliced

Directions:

In a deep saucepan, bring the water and milk to a rapid boil. Add in the oats, cover the saucepan and turn the heat to medium.

Add in the coconut sugar, vanilla and cardamom. Continue to cook for about 12 minutes, stirring periodically.

Spoon the mixture into serving bowls; top with almonds and banana. Enjoy

157) ITALIAN AROMATIC MILLET BOWL

Preparation Time: 20 minutes | | **Servings:** 3

Ingredients:

- 1 cup water
- 1 ½ cups coconut milk
- 1 cup millet, rinsed and drained
- 1/4 tsp crystallized ginger
- 1/4 tsp ground cinnamon
- A pinch of grated nutmeg
- A pinch of Himalayan salt
- 2 tbsp maple syrup

Directions:

Place the water, milk, millet, crystallized ginger cinnamon, nutmeg and salt in a saucepan; bring to a boil.

Turn the heat to a simmer and let it cook for about 20 minutes; fluff the millet with a fork and spoon into individual bowls.

Serve with maple syrup. Enjoy

158) SPICY HARISSA BULGUR BOWL

Preparation Time: 25 minutes | | **Servings:** 4

Ingredients:

- 1 cup bulgur wheat
- 1 ½ cups vegetable broth
- 2 cups sweet corn kernels, thawed
- 1 cup canned kidney beans, drained
- 1 red onion, thinly sliced
- 1 garlic clove, minced
- Sea salt and ground black pepper, to taste
- 1/4 cup harissa paste
- 1 tbsp lemon juice
- 1 tbsp white vinegar
- 1/4 cup extra-virgin olive oil
- 1/4 cup fresh parsley leaves, roughly chopped

Directions:

In a deep saucepan, bring the bulgur wheat and vegetable broth to a simmer; let it cook, covered, for 12 to 13 minutes.

Let it stand for 5 to 10 minutes and fluff your bulgur with a fork.

Add the remaining ingredients to the cooked bulgur wheat; serve warm or at room temperature. Enjoy

159) EXOTIC COCONUT QUINOA PUDDING

Preparation Time: 20 minutes | | **Servings:** 3

Ingredients:

- 1 cup water
- 1 cup coconut milk
- 1 cup quinoa
- A pinch of kosher salt
- A pinch of ground allspice
- 1/2 tsp cinnamon
- 1/2 tsp vanilla extract
- 4 tbsp agave syrup
- 1/2 cup coconut flakes

Directions:

Place the water, coconut milk, quinoa, salt, ground allspice, cinnamon and vanilla extract in a saucepan.

Bring it to a boil over medium-high heat. Turn the heat to a simmer and let it cook for about 20 minutes; fluff with a fork and add in the agave syrup.

Divide between three serving bowls and garnish with coconut flakes. Enjoy

160) ITALIAN CREMINI MUSHROOM RISOTTO

Preparation Time: 20 minutes | | **Servings:** 3

Ingredients:

- ✓ 3 tbsp vegan butter
- ✓ 1 tsp garlic, minced
- ✓ 1 tsp thyme
- ✓ 1 pound Cremini mushrooms, sliced
- ✓ 1 ½ cups white rice
- ✓ 2 ½ cups vegetable broth
- ✓ 1/4 cup dry sherry wine
- ✓ Kosher salt and ground black pepper, to taste
- ✓ 3 tbsp fresh scallions, thinly sliced

Directions:

In a saucepan, melt the vegan butter over a moderately high flame. Cook the garlic and thyme for about 1 minute or until aromatic.

Add in the mushrooms and continue to sauté until they release the liquid or about 3 minutes.

Add in the rice, vegetable broth and sherry wine. Bring to a boil; immediately turn the heat to a gentle simmer.

Cook for about 15 minutes or until all the liquid has absorbed. Fluff the rice with a fork, season with salt and pepper and garnish with fresh scallions. Enjoy

161) AUTHENTIC UKRAINIAN BORSCHT

Preparation Time: 40 minutes | | **Servings:** 4

Ingredients:

- ✓ 2 tbsp sesame oil
- ✓ 1 red onion, chopped
- ✓ 2 carrots, trimmed and sliced
- ✓ 2 large beets, peeled and sliced
- ✓ 2 large potatoes, peeled and diced
- ✓ 4 cups vegetable stock
- ✓ 2 garlic cloves, minced
- ✓ 1/2 tsp caraway seeds
- ✓ 1/2 tsp celery seeds
- ✓ 1/2 tsp fennel seeds
- ✓ 1 pound red cabbage, shredded
- ✓ 1/2 tsp mixed peppercorns, freshly cracked
- ✓ Kosher salt, to taste
- ✓ 2 bay leaves
- ✓ 2 tbsp wine vinegar

Directions:

- ❖ In a Dutch oven, heat the sesame oil over a moderate flame. Once hot, sauté the onions until tender and translucent, about 6 minutes.
- ❖ Add in the carrots, beets and potatoes and continue to sauté an additional 10 minutes, adding the vegetable stock periodically.
- ❖ Next, stir in the garlic, caraway seeds, celery seeds, fennel seeds and continue sautéing for another 30 seconds.
- ❖ Add in the cabbage, mixed peppercorns, salt and bay leaves. Add in the remaining stock and bring to boil.
- ❖ Immediately turn the heat to a simmer and continue to cook for 20 to 23 minutes longer until the vegetables have softened.
- ❖ Ladle into individual bowls and drizzle wine vinegar over it. Serve and enjoy

162) MOROCCAN LENTIL BELUGA SALAD

Preparation Time: 20 minutes + chilling time | | **Servings:** 4

Ingredients:

- ✓ 1 cup Beluga lentils, rinsed
- ✓ 1 Persian cucumber, sliced
- ✓ 1 large-sized tomatoes, sliced
- ✓ 1 red onion, chopped
- ✓ 1 bell pepper, sliced
- ✓ 1/4 cup fresh basil, chopped
- ✓ 1/4 cup fresh Italian parsley, chopped
- ✓ 2 ounces green olives, pitted and sliced
- ✓ 1/4 cup olive oil
- ✓ 4 tbsp lemon juice
- ✓ 1 tsp deli mustard
- ✓ 1/2 tsp garlic, minced
- ✓ 1/2 tsp red pepper flakes, crushed
- ✓ Sea salt and ground black pepper, to taste

Directions:

- ❖ In a large-sized saucepan, bring 3 cups of the water and 1 cup of the lentils to a boil.
- ❖ Immediately turn the heat to a simmer and continue to cook your lentils for a further 15 to 17 minutes or until they've softened but not mushy. Drain and let it cool completely.
- ❖ Transfer the lentils to a salad bowl; add in the cucumber, tomatoes, onion, pepper, basil, parsley and olives.
- ❖ In a small mixing dish, whisk the olive oil, lemon juice, mustard, garlic, red pepper, salt and black pepper.
- ❖ Dress the salad, toss to combine and serve well-chilled. Enjoy

163)   INDIAN-STYLE NAAN SALAD

Preparation Time: 10 minutes		**Servings: 3**

Ingredients:

- ✓ 3 tbsp sesame oil
- ✓ 1 tsp ginger, peeled and minced
- ✓ 1/2 tsp cumin seeds
- ✓ 1/2 tsp mustard seeds
- ✓ 1/2 tsp mixed peppercorns
- ✓ 1 tbsp curry leaves
- ✓ 3 naan breads, broken into bite-sized pieces
- ✓ 1 shallot, chopped
- ✓ 2 tomatoes, chopped
- ✓ Himalayan salt, to taste
- ✓ 1 tbsp soy sauce

Directions:

- ❖ Heat 2 tbsp of the sesame oil in a non-stick skillet over a moderately high heat.
- ❖ Sauté the ginger, cumin seeds, mustard seeds, mixed peppercorns and curry leaves for 1 minute or so, until fragrant.
- ❖ Stir in the naan breads and continue to cook, stirring periodically, until golden-brown and well coated with the spices.
- ❖ Place the shallot and tomatoes in a salad bowl; toss them with the salt, soy sauce and the remaining 1 tbsp of the sesame oil.
- ❖ Place the toasted naan on the top of your salad and serve at room temperature. Enjoy

164)   ITALIAN BROCCOLI GINGER SOUP

Preparation Time: 50 minutes		**Servings: 4**

Ingredients:

- ✓ 1 onion, chopped
- ✓ 1 tbsp minced peeled fresh ginger
- ✓ 2 tsp olive oil
- ✓ 2 carrots, chopped
- ✓ 1 head broccoli, chopped into florets
- ✓ 1 cup coconut milk
- ✓ 3 cups vegetable broth
- ✓ ½ tsp turmeric
- ✓ Salt and black pepper to taste

Directions:

- ❖ In a pot over medium heat, place the onion, ginger, and olive oil, cook for 4 minutes. Add in carrots, broccoli, broth, turmeric, pepper, and salt. Bring to a boil and cook for 15 minutes. Transfer the soup to a food processor and blend until smooth. Stir in coconut milk and serve warm

165)   ASIAN NOODLE RICE SOUP WITH BEANS

Preparation Time: 10 minutes		**Servings: 6**

Ingredients:

- ✓ 2 carrots, chopped
- ✓ 2 celery stalks, chopped
- ✓ 6 cups vegetable broth
- ✓ 8 oz brown rice noodles
- ✓ 1 (15-oz) can pinto beans
- ✓ 1 tsp dried herbs

Directions:

- ❖ Place a pot over medium heat and add in the carrots, celery, and vegetable broth. Bring to a boil. Add in noodles, beans, dried herbs, salt, and pepper. Reduce the heat and simmer for 5 minutes. Serve

166)   SPECIAL VEGETABLE AND RICE SOUP

Preparation Time: 40 minutes		**Servings: 6**

Ingredients:

- ✓ 3 tbsp olive oil
- ✓ 2 carrots, chopped
- ✓ 1 onion, chopped
- ✓ 1 celery stalk, chopped
- ✓ 2 garlic cloves, minced
- ✓ 2 cups chopped cabbage
- ✓ ½ red bell pepper, chopped
- ✓ 4 potatoes, unpeeled and quartered
- ✓ 6 cups vegetable broth
- ✓ ½ cup brown rice, rinsed
- ✓ ½ cup frozen green peas
- ✓ 2 tbsp chopped parsley

Directions:

- ❖ Heat the oil in a pot over medium heat. Place carrots, onion, celery, and garlic. Cook for 5 minutes. Add in cabbage, bell pepper, potatoes, and broth. Bring to a boil, then lower the heat and add the brown rice, salt, and pepper. Simmer uncovered for 25 minutes until vegetables are tender. Stir in peas and cook for 5 minutes. Top with parsley and serve warm

167) EASY DAIKON AND SWEET POTATO SOUP

Preparation Time: 40 minutes		Servings: 6

Ingredients:

- ✓ 6 cups water
- ✓ 2 tsp olive oil
- ✓ 1 chopped onion
- ✓ 3 garlic cloves, minced
- ✓ 1 tbsp thyme
- ✓ 2 tsp paprika
- ✓ 2 cups peeled and chopped daikon
- ✓ 2 cups chopped sweet potatoes
- ✓ 2 cups peeled and chopped parsnips
- ✓ ½ tsp sea salt
- ✓ 1 cup fresh mint, chopped
- ✓ ½ avocado
- ✓ 2 tbsp balsamic vinegar
- ✓ 2 tbsp pumpkin seeds

Directions:

❖ Heat the oil in a pot and place onion and garlic. Sauté for 3 minutes. Add in thyme, paprika, daikon, sweet potato, parsnips, water, and salt. Bring to a boil and cook for 30 minutes. Remove the soup to a food processor and add in balsamic vinegar; purée until smooth. Top with mint and pumpkin seeds to serve

168) TASTY CHICKPEA AND VEGETABLE SOUP

Preparation Time: 35 minutes		Servings: 5

Ingredients:

- ✓ 2 tbsp olive oil
- ✓ 1 onion, chopped
- ✓ 1 carrot, chopped
- ✓ 1 celery stalk, chopped
- ✓ 1 eggplant, chopped
- ✓ 1 (28-oz) can diced tomatoes
- ✓ 2 tbsp tomato paste
- ✓ 1 (15.5-oz) can chickpeas, drained
- ✓ 2 tsp smoked paprika
- ✓ 1 tsp ground cumin
- ✓ 1 tsp za'atar spice
- ✓ ¼ tsp ground cayenne pepper
- ✓ 6 cups vegetable broth
- ✓ 4 oz whole-wheat vermicelli
- ✓ 2 tbsp minced cilantro

Directions:

❖ Heat the oil in a pot over medium heat. Place onion, carrot, and celery and cook for 5 minutes. Add in eggplant, tomatoes, tomato paste, chickpeas, paprika, cumin, za´atar spice, and cayenne pepper. Stir in broth and salt. Bring to a boil, then lower the heat and simmer for 15 minutes. Add in vermicelli and cook for another 5 minutes. Serve topped with cilantro

169) ITALIAN-STYLE BEAN SOUP

Preparation Time: 1 hour 25 minutes		Servings: 6

Ingredients:

- ✓ 3 tbsp olive oil
- ✓ 2 celery stalks, chopped
- ✓ 2 carrots, chopped
- ✓ 3 shallots, chopped
- ✓ 3 garlic cloves, minced
- ✓ ½ cup brown rice
- ✓ 6 cups vegetable broth
- ✓ 1 (14.5-oz) can diced tomatoes
- ✓ 2 bay leaves
- ✓ Salt and black pepper to taste
- ✓ 2 (15.5-oz) cans white beans
- ✓ ¼ cup chopped basil

Directions:

❖ Heat oil in a pot over medium heat. Place celery, carrots, shallots, and garlic and cook for 5 minutes. Add in brown rice, broth, tomatoes, bay leaves, salt, and pepper. Bring to a boil, then lower the heat and simmer uncovered for 20 minutes. Stir in beans and basil and cook for 5 minutes. Discard bay leaves and spoon into bowls. Sprinkle with basil and serve

170)   LOVELY BRUSSELS SPROUTS AND TOFU SOUP

Preparation Time: 40 minutes | | **Servings: 4**

Ingredients:

- 7 oz firm tofu, cubed
- 2 tsp olive oil
- 1 cup sliced mushrooms
- 1 cup shredded Brussels sprouts
- 1 garlic clove, minced
- ½-inch piece fresh ginger, minced

- ✓ Salt to taste
- ✓ 2 tbsp apple cider vinegar
- ✓ 2 tbsp soy sauce
- ✓ 1 tsp pure date sugar
- ✓ ¼ tsp red pepper flakes
- ✓ 1 scallion, chopped

Directions:

- ❖ Heat the oil in a skillet over medium heat. Place mushrooms, Brussels sprouts, garlic, ginger, and salt. Sauté for 7-8 minutes until the veggies are soft. Pour in 4 cups of water, vinegar, soy sauce, sugar, pepper flakes, and tofu. Bring to a boil, then lower the heat and simmer for 5-10 minutes. Top with scallions and serve

171)   CREAMY WHITE BEAN ROSEMARY SOUP

Preparation Time: 30 minutes | | **Servings: 4**

Ingredients:

- 2 tsp olive oil
- 1 carrot, chopped
- 1 onion, chopped
- 2 garlic cloves, minced
- 1 tbsp rosemary, chopped

- ✓ 2 tbsp apple cider vinegar
- ✓ 1 cup dried white beans
- ✓ ¼ tsp salt
- ✓ 2 tbsp nutritional yeast

Directions:

- ❖ Heat the oil in a pot over medium heat. Place carrots, onion, and garlic and cook for 5 minutes.
- ❖ Pour in vinegar to deglaze the pot. Stir in 5 cups water and beans and bring to a boil. Lower the heat and simmer for 45 minutes until the beans are soft. Add in salt and nutritional yeast and stir. Serve topped with chopped rosemary

172)   DELICIOUS MUSHROOM AND TOFU SOUP

Preparation Time: 20 minutes | | **Servings: 4**

Ingredients:

- 4 cups water
- 2 tbsp soy sauce
- 4 white mushrooms, sliced

- ✓ ¼ cup chopped green onions
- ✓ 3 tbsp tahini
- ✓ 6 oz extra-firm tofu, diced

Directions:

- ❖ Pour the water and soy sauce into a pot and bring to a boil. Add in mushrooms and green onions. Lower the heat and simmer for 10 minutes. In a bowl, combine ½ cup of hot soup with tahini. Pour the mixture into the pot and simmer 2 minutes more, but not boil. Stir in tofu. Serve warm

173)   TROPICAL COCONUT CREAM BUTTERNUT SQUASH SOUP

Preparation Time: 30 minutes | | **Servings: 5**

Ingredients:

- 1 (2-lb) butternut squash, cubed
- 1 red bell pepper, chopped
- 1 large onion, chopped

- ✓ 3 garlic cloves, minced
- ✓ 4 cups vegetable broth
- ✓ 1 cup coconut cream

Directions:

- ❖ Place the squash, bell pepper, onion, garlic, and broth in a pot. Bring to a boil. Lower the heat and simmer for 20 minutes. Stir in coconut cream, salt and pepper. Transfer to a food processor purée the soup until smooth. Serve warm

174)   ITALIAN MUSHROOM COCONUT SOUP

Preparation Time: 20 minutes | | **Servings:** 2

Ingredients:

- ✓ 2 tsp olive oil
- ✓ 1 onion, chopped
- ✓ 2 garlic cloves, minced
- ✓ 2 cups chopped mushrooms
- ✓ Salt and black pepper to taste
- ✓ 2 tbsp whole-wheat flour
- ✓ 1 tsp dried rosemary
- ✓ 4 cups vegetable broth
- ✓ 1 cup coconut cream

Directions:

- ❖ In a pot over medium heat, warm the oil. Place the onion, garlic, mushrooms, and salt and cook for 5 minutes. Stir in the flour and cook for another 1-2 minutes. Add in rosemary, vegetable broth, coconut cream, and pepper. Lower the heat and simmer for 10 minutes. Serve

175)   GREEK TOMATO CREAM SOUP

Preparation Time: 15 minutes | | **Servings:** 5

Ingredients:

- ✓ 1 (28-oz) can tomatoes
- ✓ 2 tbsp olive oil
- ✓ 1 tsp smoked paprika
- ✓ 2 cups vegetable broth
- ✓ 2 tsp dried herbs
- ✓ 1 red onion, chopped
- ✓ 1 cup unsweetened non-dairy milk
- ✓ Salt and black pepper to taste

Directions:

- ❖ Place the tomatoes, olive oil, paprika, broth, dried herbs, onion, milk, salt, and pepper in a pot. Bring to a boil and cook for 10 minutes. Transfer to a food processor and blend the soup until smooth

176)   SPECIAL ROASTED PEPPER SALAD IN GREEK-STYLE

Preparation Time: 10 minutes | | **Servings:** 2

Ingredients:

- ✓ 2 red bell peppers
- ✓ 2 yellow bell peppers
- ✓ 2 garlic cloves, pressed
- ✓ 4 tsp extra-virgin olive oil
- ✓ 1 tbsp capers, rinsed and drained
- ✓ 2 tbsp red wine vinegar
- ✓ Seas salt and ground pepper, to taste
- ✓ 1 tsp fresh dill weed, chopped
- ✓ 1 tsp fresh oregano, chopped
- ✓ 1/4 cup Kalamata olives, pitted and sliced

Directions:

- ❖ Broil the peppers on a parchment-lined baking sheet for about 10 minutes, rotating the pan halfway through the cooking time, until they are charred on all sides.
- ❖ Then, cover the peppers with a plastic wrap to steam. Discard the skin, seeds and cores.
- ❖ Slice the peppers into strips and place them in a salad bowl. Add in the remaining ingredients and toss to combine well.
- ❖ Place in your refrigerator until ready to serve. Enjoy

177)   SWEET POTATO AND KIDNEY BEAN SOUP

Preparation Time: 30 minutes | | **Servings:** 4

Ingredients:

- ✓ 2 tbsp olive oil
- ✓ 1 onion, chopped
- ✓ 1 pound potatoes, peeled and diced
- ✓ 1 medium celery stalks, chopped
- ✓ 2 garlic cloves, minced
- ✓ 1 tsp paprika

- ✓ 4 cups water
- ✓ 2 tbsp vegan bouillon powder
- ✓ 16 ounces canned kidney beans, drained
- ✓ 2 cups baby spinach
- ✓ Sea salt and ground black pepper, to taste

Directions:

- ❖ In a heavy-bottomed pot, heat the olive over medium-high heat. Now, sauté the onion, potatoes and celery for approximately 5 minutes or until the onion is translucent and tender.
- ❖ Add in the garlic and continue to sauté for 1 minute or until aromatic.
- ❖ Then, add in the paprika, water and vegan bouillon powder and bring to a boil. Immediately reduce the heat to a simmer and let it cook for 15 minutes.
- ❖ Fold in the navy beans and spinach; continue to simmer for about 5 minutes until everything is thoroughly heated. Season with salt and black pepper to taste.
- ❖ Ladle into individual bowls and serve hot. Enjoy

178)   WINTER QUINOA SALAD WITH PICKLES

Preparation Time: 20 minutes + chilling time | | **Servings:** 4

Ingredients:

- ✓ 1 cup quinoa
- ✓ 4 garlic cloves, minced
- ✓ 2 pickled cucumber, chopped
- ✓ 10 ounces canned red peppers, chopped
- ✓ 1/2 cup green olives, pitted and sliced
- ✓ 2 cups green cabbages, shredded
- ✓ 2 cups Iceberg lettuce, torn into pieces

- ✓ 4 pickled chilies, chopped
- ✓ 4 tbsp olive oil
- ✓ 1 tbsp lemon juice
- ✓ 1 tsp lemon zest
- ✓ 1/2 tsp dried marjoram
- ✓ Sea salt and ground black pepper, to taste
- ✓ 1/4 cup fresh chives, coarsely chopped

Directions:

- ❖ Place two cups of water and the quinoa in a pot and bring it to a boil. Immediately turn the heat to a simmer.
- ❖ Let it simmer for about 13 minutes until the quinoa has absorbed all of the water; fluff the quinoa with a fork and let it cool completely. Then, transfer the quinoa to a salad bowl.
- ❖ Add the garlic, pickled cucumber, peppers, olives, cabbage, lettuce and pickled chilies to the salad bowl and toss to combine.
- ❖ In a small mixing bowl, make the dressing by whisking the remaining ingredients. Dress the salad, toss to combine well and serve immediately. Enjoy

179)   SUPER WILD ROASTED MUSHROOM SOUP

Preparation Time: 55 minutes | | **Servings:** 3

Ingredients:

- ✓ 3 tbsp sesame oil
- ✓ 1 pound mixed wild mushrooms, sliced
- ✓ 1 white onion, chopped
- ✓ 3 cloves garlic, minced and divided
- ✓ 2 sprigs thyme, chopped
- ✓ 2 sprigs rosemary, chopped

- ✓ 1/4 cup flaxseed meal
- ✓ 1/4 cup dry white wine
- ✓ 3 cups vegetable broth
- ✓ 1/2 tsp red chili flakes
- ✓ Garlic salt and freshly ground black pepper, to seasoned

Directions:

- ❖ Start by preheating your oven to 395 degrees F.
- ❖ Place the mushrooms in a single layer onto a parchment-lined baking pan. Drizzle the mushrooms with 1 tbsp of the sesame oil.
- ❖ Roast the mushrooms in the preheated oven for about 25 minutes, or until tender.
- ❖ Heat the remaining 2 tbsp of the sesame oil in a stockpot over medium heat. Then, sauté the onion for about 3 minutes or until tender and translucent.
- ❖ Then, add in the garlic, thyme and rosemary and continue to sauté for 1 minute or so until aromatic. Sprinkle flaxseed meal over everything.
- ❖ Add in the remaining ingredients and continue to simmer for 10 to 15 minutes longer or until everything is cooked through.
- ❖ Stir in the roasted mushrooms and continue simmering for a further 12 minutes. Ladle into soup bowls and serve hot. Enjoy

180) SPECIAL GREEN BEAN SOUP IN MEDITERRANEAN-STYLE

Preparation Time: 25 minutes		Servings: 5

Ingredients:

- ✓ 2 tbsp olive oil
- ✓ 1 onion, chopped
- ✓ 1 celery with leaves, chopped
- ✓ 1 carrot, chopped
- ✓ 2 garlic cloves, minced
- ✓ 1 zucchini, chopped
- ✓ 5 cups vegetable broth

- ✓ 1 ¼ pounds green beans, trimmed and cut into bite-sized chunks
- ✓ 2 medium-sized tomatoes, pureed
- ✓ Sea salt and freshly ground black pepper, to taste
- ✓ 1/2 tsp cayenne pepper
- ✓ 1 tsp oregano
- ✓ 1/2 tsp dried dill
- ✓ 1/2 cup Kalamata olives, pitted and sliced

Directions:

- ❖ In a heavy-bottomed pot, heat the olive over medium-high heat. Now, sauté the onion, celery and carrot for about 4 minutes or until the vegetables are just tender.
- ❖ Add in the garlic and zucchini and continue to sauté for 1 minute or until aromatic.
- ❖ Then, stir in the vegetable broth, green beans, tomatoes, salt, black pepper, cayenne pepper, oregano and dried dill; bring to a boil. Immediately reduce the heat to a simmer and let it cook for about 15 minutes.
- ❖ Ladle into individual bowls and serve with sliced olives. Enjoy

181) LOVELY CREAMY CARROT SOUP

Preparation Time: 30 minutes		Servings: 4

Ingredients:

- ✓ 2 tbsp sesame oil
- ✓ 1 onion, chopped
- ✓ 1 ½ pounds carrots, trimmed and chopped
- ✓ 1 parsnip, chopped
- ✓ 2 garlic cloves, minced

- ✓ 1/2 tsp curry powder
- ✓ Sea salt and cayenne pepper, to taste
- ✓ 4 cups vegetable broth
- ✓ 1 cup full-fat coconut milk

Directions:

- ❖ In a heavy-bottomed pot, heat the sesame oil over medium-high heat. Now, sauté the onion, carrots and parsnip for about 5 minutes, stirring periodically.
- ❖ Add in the garlic and continue sautéing for 1 minute or until fragrant.
- ❖ Then, stir in the curry powder, salt, cayenne pepper and vegetable broth; bring to a rapid boil. Immediately reduce the heat to a simmer and let it cook for 18 to 20 minutes.
- ❖ Puree the soup using an immersion blender until creamy and uniform.
- ❖ Return the pureed mixture to the pot. Fold in the coconut milk and continue to simmer until heated through or about 5 minutes longer.
- ❖ Ladle into four bowls and serve hot. Enjoy

182) SPECIAL ITALIAN NONNO'S PIZZA SALAD

Preparation Time: 15 minutes + chilling time		Servings: 4

Ingredients:

- ✓ 1 pound macaroni
- ✓ 1 cup marinated mushrooms, sliced
- ✓ 1 cup grape tomatoes, halved
- ✓ 4 tbsp scallions, chopped
- ✓ 1 tsp garlic, minced
- ✓ 1 Italian pepper, sliced

- ✓ 1/4 cup extra-virgin olive oil
- ✓ 1/4 cup balsamic vinegar
- ✓ 1 tsp dried oregano
- ✓ 1 tsp dried basil
- ✓ 1/2 tsp dried rosemary
- ✓ Sea salt and cayenne pepper, to taste
- ✓ 1/2 cup black olives, sliced

Directions:

- ❖ Cook the pasta according to the package directions. Drain and rinse the pasta. Let it cool completely and then, transfer it to a salad bowl.
- ❖ Then, add in the remaining ingredients and toss until the macaroni are well coated.
- ❖ Taste and adjust the seasonings; place the pizza salad in your refrigerator until ready to use. Enjoy

183)   SPECIAL CREAM OF GOLDEN VEGGIE SOUP

Preparation Time: 45 minutes		Servings: 4

Ingredients:

- ✓ 2 tbsp avocado oil
- ✓ 1 yellow onion, chopped
- ✓ 2 Yukon Gold potatoes, peeled and diced
- ✓ 2 pounds butternut squash, peeled, seeded and diced
- ✓ 1 parsnip, trimmed and sliced
- ✓ 1 tsp ginger-garlic paste

- ✓ 1 tsp turmeric powder
- ✓ 1 tsp fennel seeds
- ✓ 1/2 tsp chili powder
- ✓ 1/2 tsp pumpkin pie spice
- ✓ Kosher salt and ground black pepper, to taste
- ✓ 3 cups vegetable stock
- ✓ 1 cup full-fat coconut milk
- ✓ 2 tbsp pepitas

Directions:

- ❖ In a heavy-bottomed pot, heat the oil over medium-high heat. Now, sauté the onion, potatoes, butternut squash and parsnip for about 10 minutes, stirring periodically to ensure even cooking.
- ❖ Add in the ginger-garlic paste and continue sautéing for 1 minute or until aromatic.
- ❖ Then, stir in the turmeric powder, fennel seeds, chili powder, pumpkin pie spice, salt, black pepper and vegetable stock; bring to a boil. Immediately reduce the heat to a simmer and let it cook for about 25 minutes.
- ❖ Puree the soup using an immersion blender until creamy and uniform.
- ❖ Return the pureed mixture to the pot. Fold in the coconut milk and continue to simmer until heated through or about 5 minutes longer.
- ❖ Ladle into individual bowls and serve garnished with pepitas. Enjoy

184)   EASY ROASTED CAULIFLOWER SOUP

Preparation Time: 1 hour		Servings: 4

Ingredients:

- ✓ 1 ½ pounds cauliflower florets
- ✓ 4 tbsp olive oil
- ✓ 1 onion, chopped
- ✓ 2 cloves garlic, minced
- ✓ 1/2 tsp ginger, peeled and minced
- ✓ 1 tsp fresh rosemary, chopped

- ✓ 2 tbsp fresh basil, chopped
- ✓ 2 tbsp fresh parsley, chopped
- ✓ 4 cups vegetable stock
- ✓ Sea salt and ground black pepper, to taste
- ✓ 1/2 tsp ground sumac
- ✓ 1/4 cup tahini
- ✓ 1 lemon, freshly squeezed

Directions:

- ❖ Begin by preheating the oven to 425 degrees F. Toss the cauliflower with 2 tbsp of the olive oil and arrange them on a parchment-lined roasting pan.
- ❖ Then, roast the cauliflower florets for about 30 minutes stirring, them once or twice to promote even cooking.
- ❖ Meanwhile, in a heavy-bottomed pot, heat the remaining 2 tbsp of the olive oil over medium-high heat. Now, sauté the onion for about 4 minutes until tender and translucent.
- ❖ Add in the garlic, ginger, rosemary, basil and parsley and continue sautéing for 1 minute or until fragrant.
- ❖ Then, stir in the vegetable stock, salt, black pepper and sumac and bring it to a boil. Immediately reduce the heat to a simmer and let it cook for about 20 to 22 minutes.
- ❖ Puree the soup using an immersion blender until creamy and uniform.
- ❖ Return the pureed mixture to the pot. Fold in the tahini and continue to simmer for about 5 minutes or until everything is thoroughly cooked.
- ❖ Ladle into individual bowls, garnish with lemon juice and serve hot. Enjoy

185) AUTHENTIC VEGAN COLESLAW

Preparation Time: 10 minutes		Servings: 4

Ingredients:

- ✓ 1 pound red cabbage, shredded
- ✓ 2 carrots, trimmed and grated
- ✓ 4 tbsp onion, chopped
- ✓ 1 garlic clove, minced
- ✓ 1/2 cup fresh Italian parsley, roughly chopped
- ✓ 1 cup vegan mayo
- ✓ 1 tsp brown mustard
- ✓ 1 tsp lemon zest
- ✓ 2 tbsp apple cider vinegar
- ✓ Sea salt and ground black pepper, to taste
- ✓ 2 tbsp sunflower seeds

Directions:

- ❖ Toss the cabbage, carrots, onion, garlic and parsley in a salad bowl.
- ❖ In a mixing bowl, whisk the mayo, mustard, lemon zest, apple cider vinegar, salt and black pepper.
- ❖ Dress your salad and serve garnished with the sunflower seeds

186) SUPER HOT COLLARD SALAD

Preparation Time: 10 minutes		Servings: 2

Ingredients:

- ✓ ¾ cup coconut whipping cream
- ✓ 2 tbsp tofu mayonnaise
- ✓ A pinch of mustard powder
- ✓ 2 tbsp coconut oil
- ✓ 1 garlic clove, minced
- ✓ Salt and black pepper to taste
- ✓ 2 oz plant butter
- ✓ 1 cup collards, rinsed
- ✓ 4 oz tofu cheese

Directions:

- ❖ In a small bowl, whisk the coconut whipping cream, tofu mayonnaise, mustard powder, coconut oil, garlic, salt, and black pepper until well mixed; set aside. Melt the plant butter in a large skillet over medium heat and sauté the collards until wilted and brownish. Season with salt and black pepper to taste. Transfer the collards to a salad bowl and pour the creamy dressing over. Mix the salad well and crumble the tofu cheese over. Serve

187) SUPER ROASTED MUSHROOMS AND GREEN BEANS SALAD

Preparation Time: 25 minutes		Servings: 4

Ingredients:

- ✓ 1 lb. cremini mushrooms, sliced
- ✓ ½ cup green beans
- ✓ 3 tbsp melted plant butter
- ✓ Salt and black pepper to taste
- ✓ Juice of 1 lemon
- ✓ 4 tbsp toasted hazelnuts

Directions:

- ❖ Preheat oven to 450 F.
- ❖ Arrange the mushrooms and green beans in a baking dish, drizzle the plant butter over, and sprinkle with salt and black pepper. Use your hands to rub the vegetables with the seasoning and roast in the oven for 20 minutes or until they are soft. Transfer the vegetables into a salad bowl, drizzle with the lemon juice, and toss the salad with the hazelnuts. Serve the salad immediately

188) MEXICAN BEAN AND COUSCOUS SALAD

Preparation Time: 15 minutes		Servings: 4

Ingredients:

- ✓ ¼ cup olive oil
- ✓ 1 medium shallot, minced
- ✓ ½ tsp ground coriander
- ✓ ½ tsp turmeric
- ✓ ¼ tsp ground cayenne
- ✓ 1 cup couscous
- ✓ 2 cups vegetable broth
- ✓ 1 yellow bell pepper, chopped
- ✓ 1 carrot, shredded
- ✓ ½ cup chopped dried apricots
- ✓ ¼ cup golden raisins
- ✓ ¼ cup chopped roasted cashews
- ✓ 1 (15.5-oz) can white beans
- ✓ 2 tbsp minced fresh cilantro leaves
- ✓ 2 tbsp fresh lemon juice

Directions:

- ❖ Heat 1 tbsp of oil in a pot over medium heat. Place in shallot, coriander, turmeric, cayenne pepper, and couscous. Cook for 2 minutes, stirring often. Add in broth and salt. Bring to a boil. Turn the heat off and let sit covered for 5 minutes. Remove to a bowl and stir in bell pepper, carrot, apricots, raisins, cashews, beans, and cilantro. Set aside. In another bowl, whisk the remaining oil with lemon juice until blended. Pour over the salad and toss to combine. Serve immediately

189) VEGETARIAN SEITAN AND SPINACH SALAD A LA PUTTANESCA

Preparation Time: 11 minutes | | **Servings:** 4

Ingredients:

- ✓ 4 tbsp olive oil
- ✓ 8 oz seitan, cut into strips
- ✓ 2 garlic cloves, minced
- ✓ ½ cup Kalamata olives, halved
- ✓ ½ cup green olives, halved
- ✓ 2 tbsp capers
- ✓ 3 cups baby spinach, cut into strips
- ✓ 1 ½ cups cherry tomatoes, halved
- ✓ 2 tbsp balsamic vinegar
- ✓ 2 tbsp torn fresh basil leaves
- ✓ 2 tbsp minced fresh parsley
- ✓ 1 cup pomegranate seeds

Directions:

- ❖ Heat half of the olive oil in a skillet over medium heat. Place the seitan and brown for 5 minutes on all sides. Add in garlic and cook for 30 seconds. Remove to a bowl and let cool. Stir in olives, capers, spinach, and tomatoes. Set aside.
- ❖ In another bowl, whisk the remaining oil, vinegar, salt, and pepper until well mixed. Pour this dressing over the seitan salad and toss to coat. Top with basil, parsley, and pomegranate seeds. Serve

190) POMODORO AND AVOCADO LETTUCE SALAD

Preparation Time: 15 minutes | | **Servings:** 4

Ingredients:

- ✓ 1 garlic clove, chopped
- ✓ 1 red onion, sliced
- ✓ ½ tsp dried basil
- ✓ Salt and black pepper to taste
- ✓ ¼ tsp pure date sugar
- ✓ 3 tbsp white wine vinegar
- ✓ 1/3 cup olive oil
- ✓ 1 head Iceberg lettuce, shredded
- ✓ 12 ripe grape tomatoes, halved
- ✓ ½ cup frozen peas, thawed
- ✓ 8 black olives, pitted
- ✓ 1 avocado, sliced

Directions:

- ❖ In a food processor, place the garlic, onion, oil, basil, salt, pepper, sugar, and vinegar. Blend until smooth. Set aside. Place the lettuce, tomatoes, peas, and olives on a nice serving plate. Top with avocado slices and drizzle the previously prepared dressing all over. Serve

191) SPECIAL FRIED BROCCOLI SALAD WITH TEMPEH AND CRANBERRIES

Preparation Time: 15 minutes | | **Servings:** 4

Ingredients:

- ✓ 3 oz plant butter
- ✓ ¾ lb tempeh slices, cubed
- ✓ 1 lb broccoli florets
- ✓ Salt and black pepper to taste
- ✓ 2 oz almonds
- ✓ ½ cup frozen cranberries

Directions:

- ❖ In a skillet, melt the plant butter over medium heat until no longer foaming, and fry the tempeh cubes until brown on all sides. Add the broccoli and stir-fry for 6 minutes. Season with salt and pepper. Turn the heat off. Stir in the almonds and cranberries to warm through. Share salad into bowls and serve

192) HEALTHY BALSAMIC LENTIL SALAD

Preparation Time: 40 minutes | | **Servings:** 4

Ingredients:

- 2 tsp olive oil
- 1 red onion, diced
- 1 garlic clove, minced
- 1 carrot, diced
- 1 cup lentils
- 1 tbsp dried basil
- 1 tbsp dried oregano
- 1 tbsp balsamic vinegar
- 2 cups water
- Sea salt to taste
- 2 cups chopped Swiss chard
- 2 cups torn curly endive

Directions:

- ❖ In a bowl, mix the balsamic vinegar, olive oil, and salt. Set aside. Warm 1 tsp of oil in a pot over medium heat. Place the onion and carrot and cook for 5 minutes. Mix in lentils, basil, oregano, balsamic vinegar, and water and bring to a boil. Lower the heat and simmer for 20 minutes.
- ❖ Mix in two-thirds of the dressing. Add in the Swiss chard and cook for 5 minutes on low. Let cool. Coat the endive with the remaining dressing. Transfer to a plate and top with lentil mixture to serve

193) SUPER HOT GREEN BEAN AND POTATO SALAD

Preparation Time: 25 minutes | | **Servings:** 4

Ingredients:

- Salt and black pepper to taste
- 1 cup green beans, chopped
- 4 potatoes, quartered
- 2 carrots, sliced
- 1 tbsp extra-virgin olive oil
- 1 tbsp lime juice
- 2 tsp dried dill
- 1 cup cashew cream

Directions:

- ❖ Pour salted water in a pot over medium heat. Add in potatoes, bring to a boil and cook for 8 minutes. Put in carrots and green beans and cook for 8 minutes. Drain and put in a bowl. Mix in olive oil, lime juice, dill, cashew cream, salt, and pepper. Toss to coat. Allow cooling before serving

194) EASY MILLET SALAD WITH OLIVES AND CHERRIES

Preparation Time: 40 minutes | | **Servings:** 4

Ingredients:

- 1 cup millet
- 1 (15.5-oz) can navy beans
- 1 celery stalk, finely chopped
- 1 carrot, shredded
- 3 green onions, minced
- ½ cup chopped kalamata olives
- ½ cup dried cherries
- ½ cup toasted pecans, chopped
- ½ cup minced fresh parsley
- 1 garlic clove, pressed
- 3 tbsp sherry vinegar
- ¼ cup grapeseed oil

Directions:

- ❖ Cook the millet in salted water for 30 minutes. Remove to a bowl. Mix in beans, celery, carrot, green onions, olives, cherries, pecans, and parsley. Set aside. In another bowl, whisk the garlic, vinegar, salt, and pepper until well mixed. Pour over the millet mixture and toss to coat. Serve immediately

195) DELICIOUS DAIKON SALAD WITH CARAMELIZED ONION

Preparation Time: 50 minutes | | **Servings:** 4

Ingredients:

- 1 lb daikon, peeled
- 2 cups sliced sweet onions
- 2 tsp olive oil
- Salt to taste
- 1 tbsp rice vinegar

Directions:

- ❖ Place the daikon in a pot with salted water and cook 25 minutes, until tender. Drain and let cool. In a skillet over low heat, warm olive oil and add the onion. Sauté for 10-15 minutes until caramelized. Sprinkle with salt. Remove to a bowl. Chop the daikon into wedges and add to the onion bowl. Stir in the vinegar. Serve

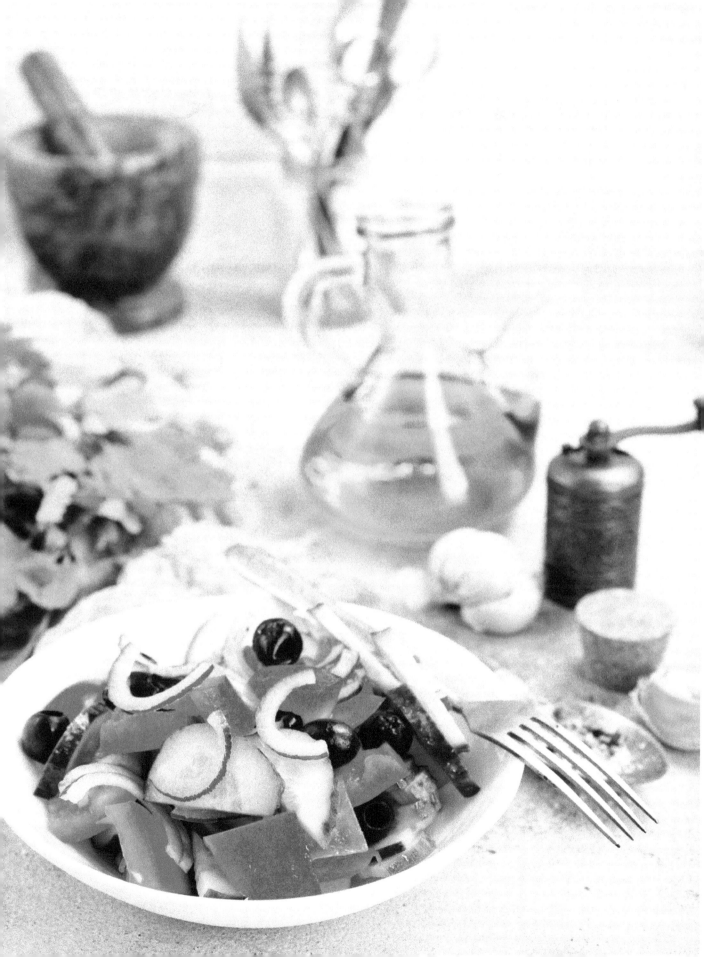

Chapter 4. DESSERTS

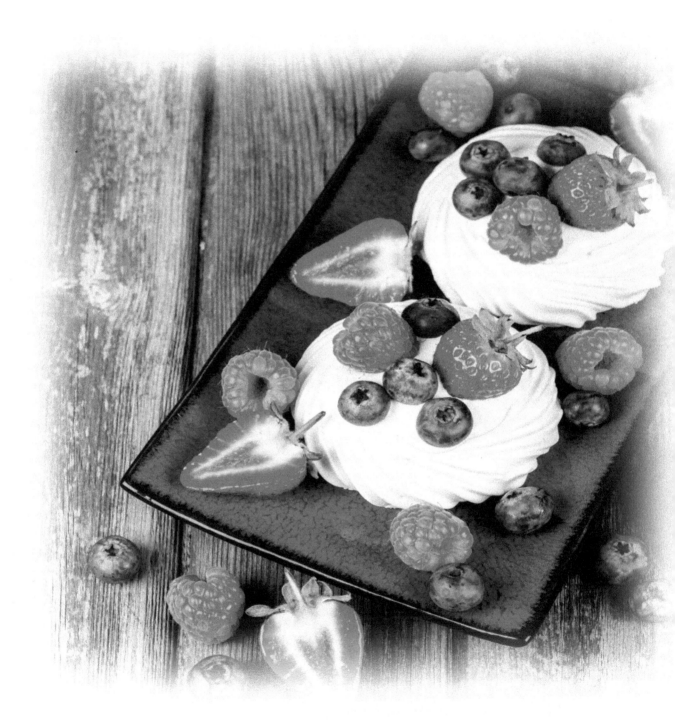

196) DELICIOUS VANILLA BROWNIES

Preparation Time: 30 minutes + chilling time		Servings: 4

Ingredients:

- ✓ 2 tbsp flaxseed powder
- ✓ ¼ cup cocoa powder
- ✓ ½ cup almond flour
- ✓ ½ tsp baking powder
- ✓ ½ cup erythritol
- ✓ 10 tbsp plant butter
- ✓ 2 oz dairy-free dark chocolate
- ✓ ½ tsp vanilla extract

Directions:

Preheat oven to 375 F and line a baking sheet with parchment paper. Mix the flaxseed powder with 6 tbsp water in a bowl and allow thickening for 5 minutes. In a separate bowl, mix cocoa powder, almond flour, baking powder, and erythritol until no lumps. In another bowl, add the plant butter and dark chocolate and melt both in the microwave for 30 seconds to 1 minute.

Whisk the vegan "flax egg" and vanilla into the chocolate mixture, then pour the mixture into the dry ingredients. Combine evenly. Pour the batter onto the paper-lined baking sheet and bake for 20 minutes. Cool completely and refrigerate for 2 hours. When ready, slice into squares and serve

197) SPEICAL VEGAN CHEESECAKE WITH BLUEBERRIES

Preparation Time: 1 hour 30 minutes + chilling time		Servings: 6

Ingredients:

- ✓ 2 oz plant butter
- ✓ 1 ¼ cups almond flour
- ✓ 3 tbsp Swerve sugar
- ✓ 1 tsp vanilla extract
- ✓ 3 tbsp flaxseed powder
- ✓ 2 cups cashew cream cheese
- ✓ ½ cup coconut cream
- ✓ 1 tsp lemon zest
- ✓ 2 oz fresh blueberries

Directions:

Preheat oven to 350 F and grease a springform pan with cooking spray. Line with parchment paper.

To make the crust, melt the plant butter in a skillet over low heat until nutty in flavor. Turn the heat off and stir in almond flour, 2 tbsp of Swerve sugar, and half of the vanilla until a dough forms. Press the mixture into the springform pan and bake for 8 minutes.

Mix flaxseed powder with 9 tbsp water and allow sitting for 5 minutes to thicken. In a bowl, combine cashew cream cheese, coconut cream, remaining Swerve sugar, lemon zest, remaining vanilla extract, and vegan "flax egg." Remove the crust from the oven and pour the mixture on top. Use a spatula to layer evenly. Bake the cake for 15 minutes at 400 F. Then, reduce the heat to 230 F and bake for 45-60 minutes. Remove to cool completely. Refrigerate overnight and scatter the blueberries on top. Serve

198) FROZEN LIME AVOCADO ICE CREAM

Preparation Time: 10 minutes		Servings: 4

Ingredients:

- ✓ 2 large avocados, pitted
- ✓ Juice and zest of 3 limes
- ✓ 1/3 cup erythritol
- ✓ 1 ¾ cups coconut cream
- ✓ ¼ tsp vanilla extract

Directions:

In a blender, combine the avocado pulp, lime juice and zest, erythritol, coconut cream, and vanilla extract. Process until the mixture is smooth. Pour the mixture into your ice cream maker and freeze based on the manufacturer's instructions. When ready, remove and scoop the ice cream into bowls. Serve immediately

199) EASY WALNUT CHOCOLATE SQUARES

Preparation Time: 10 minutes		Servings: 6

Ingredients:

- ✓ 3½ oz dairy-free dark chocolate
- ✓ 4 tbsp plant butter
- ✓ 1 pinch salt
- ✓ ¼ cup walnut butter
- ✓ ½ tsp vanilla extract
- ✓ ¼ cup chopped walnuts to garnish

Directions:

Pour the chocolate and plant butter in a safe microwave bowl and melt in the microwave for about 1 to 2 minutes. Remove the bowl from the microwave and mix in the salt, walnut butter, and vanilla.

Grease a small baking sheet with cooking spray and line with parchment paper. Pour in the batter and use a spatula to spread out into a 4 x 6-inch rectangle. Top with the chopped walnuts and chill in the refrigerator. Once set, cut into 1 x 1-inch squares. Serve while firming

200) DELICIOUS VANILLA WHITE CHOCOLATE PUDDING

Preparation Time: 20 minutes+ cooling time		Servings: 4

Ingredients:

- ✓ 3 tbsp flaxseed + 9 tbsp water
- ✓ 3 tbsp corn-starch
- ✓ 1 cup cashew cream
- ✓ 2 ½ cups almond milk
- ✓ ½ pure date sugar
- ✓ 1 tbsp vanilla caviar
- ✓ 6 oz white chocolate chips
- ✓ Whipped coconut cream
- ✓ Sliced bananas and raspberries

Directions:

In a small bowl, mix the flaxseed powder with water and allow thickening for 5 minutes to make the vegan "flax egg." In a large bowl, whisk the corn-starch and cashew cream until smooth. Beat in the vegan "flax egg" until well combined.

Pour the almond milk into a pot and whisk in the date sugar. Cook over medium heat while frequently stirring until the sugar dissolves. Reduce the heat to low and simmer until steamy and bubbly around the edges.

Pour half of the almond milk mixture into the vegan "flax egg" mix, whisk well and pour this mixture into the remaining milk content in the pot. Whisk continuously until well combined. Bring the new mixture to a boil over medium heat while still frequently stirring and scraping all the pot's corners, 2 minutes.

Turn the heat off, stir in the vanilla caviar, then the white chocolate chips until melted. Spoon the mixture into a bowl, allow cooling for 2 minutes, cover with plastic wraps, making sure to press the plastic onto the surface of the pudding, and refrigerate for 4 hours. Remove the pudding from the fridge, take off the plastic wrap, and whip for about a minute. Spoon the dessert into serving cups, swirl some coconut whipping cream on top, and top with the bananas and raspberries. Enjoy

201) TRADITIONAL GRANDMA'S APRICOT TARTE TATIN

Preparation Time: 30 minutes + cooling time		Servings: 4

Ingredients:

- ✓ 4 tbsp flaxseed powder
- ✓ ¼ cup almond flour
- ✓ 3 tbsp whole-wheat flour
- ✓ ½ tsp salt
- ✓ ¼ cup cold plant butter, crumbled
- ✓ 3 tbsp pure maple syrup
- ✓ 4 tbsp melted plant butter
- ✓ 3 tsp pure maple syrup
- ✓ 1 tsp vanilla extract
- ✓ 1 lemon, juiced
- ✓ 12 apricots, halved and pitted
- ✓ ½ cup coconut cream
- ✓ 4 fresh basil leaves

Directions:

Preheat the oven to 350 F and grease a large pie pan with cooking spray.

In a medium bowl, mix the flaxseed powder with 12 tbsp water and allow thickening for 5 minutes.

In a large bowl, combine the flours and salt. Add the plant butter and using an electric hand mixer, whisk until crumbly. Pour in the vegan "flax egg" and maple syrup and mix until smooth dough forms. Flatten the dough on a flat surface, cover with plastic wrap, and refrigerate for 1 hour.

Dust a working surface with almond flour, remove the dough onto the surface, and using a rolling pin, flatten the dough into a 1-inch diameter circle. Set aside. In a large bowl, mix the plant butter, maple syrup, vanilla, and lemon juice. Add the apricots to the mixture and coat well.

Arrange the apricots (open side down) in the pie pan and lay the dough on top. Press to fit and cut off the dough hanging on the edges. Brush the top with more plant butter and bake in the oven for 35 to 40 minutes or until golden brown and puffed up.

Remove the pie pan from the oven, allow cooling for 5 minutes, and run a butter knife around the edges of the pastry. Invert the dessert onto a large plate, spread the coconut cream on top, and garnish with the basil leaves. Slice and serve

202) AMERICAN PEANUT BUTTER OATMEAL BARS

Preparation Time: 25 minutes		Servings: 20

Ingredients:

- ✓ 1 cup vegan butter
- ✓ 3/4 cup coconut sugar
- ✓ 2 tbsp applesauce
- ✓ 1 ¾ cups old-fashioned oats
- ✓ 1 tsp baking soda
- ✓ A pinch of sea salt
- ✓ A pinch of grated nutmeg
- ✓ 1 tsp pure vanilla extract
- ✓ 1 cup oat flour
- ✓ 1 cup all-purpose flour

Directions:

Begin by preheating your oven to 350 degrees F.

In a mixing bowl, thoroughly combine the dry ingredients. In another bowl, combine the wet ingredients.

Then, stir the wet mixture into the dry ingredients; mix to combine well.

Spread the batter mixture in a parchment-lined square baking pan. Bake in the preheated oven for about 20 minutes. Enjoy

203) SPECIAL VANILLA HALVAH FUDGE

Preparation Time: 10 minutes + chilling time		Servings: 16

Ingredients:

- ✓ 1/2 cup cocoa butter
- ✓ 1/2 cup tahini
- ✓ 8 dates, pitted
- ✓ 1/4 tsp ground cloves
- ✓ A pinch of grated nutmeg
- ✓ A pinch coarse salt
- ✓ 1 tsp vanilla extract

Directions:

Line a square baking pan with parchment paper.

Mix the ingredients until everything is well incorporated.

Scrape the batter into the parchment-lined pan. Place in your freezer until ready to serve. Enjoy

204) HEALTHY RAW CHOCOLATE MANGO PIE

Preparation Time: 10 minutes + chilling time		Servings: 16

Ingredients:

- ✓ Avocado layer:
- ✓ 3 ripe avocados, pitted and peeled
- ✓ A pinch of sea salt
- ✓ A pinch of ground anise
- ✓ 1/2 tsp vanilla paste
- ✓ 2 tbsp coconut milk
- ✓ 5 tbsp agave syrup

- ✓ 1/3 cup cocoa powder
- ✓ Crema layer:
- ✓ 1/3 cup almond butter
- ✓ 1/2 cup coconut cream
- ✓ 1 medium mango, peeled
- ✓ 1/2 coconut flakes
- ✓ 2 tbsp agave syrup

Directions:

In your food processor, blend the avocado layer until smooth and uniform, reserve.

Then, blend the other layer in a separate bowl. Spoon the layers in a lightly oiled baking pan.

Transfer the cake to your freezer for about 3 hours. Store in your freezer. Enjoy

205) FROZEN CHOCOLATE N'ICE CREAM

Preparation Time: 10 minutes		Servings: 1

Ingredients:

- ✓ 2 frozen bananas, peeled and sliced
- ✓ 2 tbsp coconut milk
- ✓ 1 tsp carob powder
- ✓ 1 tsp cocoa powder

- ✓ A pinch of grated nutmeg
- ✓ 1/8 tsp ground cardamom
- ✓ 1/8 tsp ground cinnamon
- ✓ 1 tbsp chocolate curls

Directions:

Place all the ingredients in the bowl of your food processor or high-speed blender.

Blitz the ingredients until creamy or until your desired consistency is achieved.

Serve immediately or store in your freezer.

Enjoy

206) SUMMER RAW RASPBERRY CHEESECAKE

Preparation Time: 15 minutes + chilling time		Servings: 9

Ingredients:

- ✓ Crust:
- ✓ 2 cups almonds
- ✓ 1 cup fresh dates, pitted
- ✓ 1/4 tsp ground cinnamon

- ✓ Filling:
- ✓ 2 cups raw cashews, soaked overnight and drained
- ✓ 14 ounces blackberries, frozen
- ✓ 1 tbsp fresh lime juice
- ✓ 1/4 tsp crystallized ginger
- ✓ 1 can coconut cream
- ✓ 8 fresh dates, pitted

Directions:

In your food processor, blend the crust ingredients until the mixture comes together; press the crust into a lightly oiled springform pan.

Then, blend the filling layer until completely smooth. Spoon the filling onto the crust, creating a flat surface with a spatula.

Transfer the cake to your freezer for about 3 hours. Store in your freezer.

Garnish with organic citrus peel. Enjoy

207) EASY MINI LEMON TARTS

Preparation Time: 15 minutes + chilling time | | **Servings:** 9

Ingredients:

- 1 cup cashews
- 1 cup dates, pitted
- 1/2 cup coconut flakes
- 1/2 tsp anise, ground
- 3 lemons, freshly squeezed
- 1 cup coconut cream
- 2 tbsp agave syrup

Directions:

Brush a muffin tin with a nonstick cooking oil.

Blend the cashews, dates, coconut and anise in your food processor or a high-speed blender. Press the crust into the peppered muffin tin.

Then, blend the lemon, coconut cream and agave syrup. Spoon the cream into the muffin tin.

Store in your freezer. Enjoy

208) EXOTIC COCONUT BLONDIES WITH RAISINS

Preparation Time: 30 minutes | | **Servings:** 9

Ingredients:

- 1 cup coconut flour
- 1 cup all-purpose flour
- 1/2 tsp baking powder
- 1/4 tsp salt
- 1 cup desiccated coconut, unsweetened
- 3/4 cup vegan butter, softened
- 1 ½ cups brown sugar
- 3 tbsp applesauce
- 1/2 tsp vanilla extract
- 1/2 tsp ground anise
- 1 cup raisins, soaked for 15 minutes

Directions:

Start by preheating your oven to 350 degrees F. Brush a baking pan with a nonstick cooking oil.

Thoroughly combine the flour, baking powder, salt and coconut. In another bowl, mix the butter, sugar, applesauce, vanilla and anise. Stir the butter mixture into the dry ingredients; stir to combine well.

Fold in the raisins. Press the batter into the prepared baking pan.

Bake for approximately 25 minutes or until it is set in the middle. Place the cake on a wire rack to cool slightly.

Enjoy

209) SIMPLE CHOCOLATE SQUARES

Preparation Time: 1 hour 10 minutes | | **Servings:** 20

Ingredients:

- 1 cup cashew butter
- 1 cup almond butter
- 1/4 cup coconut oil, melted
- 1/4 cup raw cacao powder
- 2 ounces dark chocolate
- 4 tbsp agave syrup
- 1 tsp vanilla paste
- 1/4 tsp ground cinnamon
- 1/4 tsp ground cloves

Directions:

Process all the ingredients in your blender until uniform and smooth.

Scrape the batter into a parchment-lined baking sheet. Place it in your freezer for at least 1 hour to set.

Cut into squares and serve. Enjoy

210) DELICIOUS CHOCOLATE AND RAISIN COOKIE BARS

Preparation Time: 40 minutes | | **Servings:** 10

Ingredients:

- ✓ 1/2 cup peanut butter, at room temperature
- ✓ 1 cup agave syrup
- ✓ 1 tsp pure vanilla extract
- ✓ 1/4 tsp kosher salt
- ✓ 2 cups almond flour
- ✓ 1 tsp baking soda
- ✓ 1 cup raisins
- ✓ 1 cup vegan chocolate, broken into chunks

Directions:

In a mixing bowl, thoroughly combine the peanut butter, agave syrup, vanilla and salt.

Gradually stir in the almond flour and baking soda and stir to combine. Add in the raisins and chocolate chunks and stir again.

Freeze for about 30 minutes and serve well chilled. Enjoy

211) TASTY ALMOND GRANOLA BARS

Preparation Time: 25 minutes | | **Servings:** 12

Ingredients:

- ✓ 1/2 cup spelt flour
- ✓ 1/2 cup oat flour
- ✓ 1 cup rolled oats
- ✓ 1 tsp baking powder
- ✓ 1/2 tsp cinnamon
- ✓ 1/2 tsp ground cardamom
- ✓ 1/4 tsp freshly grated nutmeg
- ✓ 1/8 tsp kosher salt
- ✓ 1 cup almond milk
- ✓ 3 tbsp agave syrup
- ✓ 1/2 cup peanut butter
- ✓ 1/2 cup applesauce
- ✓ 1/2 tsp pure almond extract
- ✓ 1/2 tsp pure vanilla extract
- ✓ 1/2 cup almonds, slivered

Directions:

Begin by preheating your oven to 350 degrees F.

In a mixing bowl, thoroughly combine the flour, oats, baking powder and spices. In another bowl, combine the wet ingredients.

Then, stir the wet mixture into the dry ingredients; mix to combine well. Fold in the slivered almonds.

Scrape the batter mixture into a parchment-lined baking pan. Bake in the preheated oven for about 20 minutes. Let it cool on a wire rack. Cut into bars and enjoy

212) TROPICAL COCONUT COOKIES

Preparation Time: 40 minutes | | **Servings:** 10

Ingredients:

- ✓ 1/2 cup oat flour
- ✓ 1/2 cup all-purpose flour
- ✓ 1/2 tsp baking soda
- ✓ A pinch of salt
- ✓ 1/4 tsp grated nutmeg
- ✓ 1/2 tsp ground cloves
- ✓ 1/2 tsp ground cinnamon
- ✓ 4 tbsp coconut oil
- ✓ 2 tbsp oat milk
- ✓ 1/2 cup coconut sugar
- ✓ 1/2 cup coconut flakes, unsweetened

Directions:

In a mixing bowl, combine the flour, baking soda and spices.

In another bowl, combine the coconut oil, oat milk, sugar and coconut. Stir the wet mixture into the dry ingredients and stir until well combined.

Place the batter in your refrigerator for about 30 minutes. Shape the batter into small cookies and arrange them on a parchment-lined cookie pan.

Bake in the preheated oven at 330 degrees F for approximately 10 minutes. Transfer the pan to a wire rack to cool at room temperature. Enjoy

213)   HEALTHY RAW WALNUT AND BERRY CAKE

Preparation Time: 10 minutes + chilling time		Servings: 8

Ingredients:	✓ Berry layer:	Directions:
✓ Crust:	✓ 6 cups mixed berries	In your food processor, blend the crust ingredients until the mixture comes together; press the crust into a lightly oiled baking pan.
✓ 1 ½ cups walnuts, ground	✓ 2 frozen bananas	Then, blend the berry layer. Spoon the berry layer onto the crust, creating a flat surface with a spatula.
✓ 2 tbsp maple syrup	✓ 1/2 cup agave syrup	Transfer the cake to your freezer for about 3 hours. Store in your freezer. Enjoy
✓ 1/4 cup raw cacao powder		
✓ 1/4 tsp ground cinnamon		
✓ A pinch of coarse salt		
✓ A pinch of freshly grated nutmeg		

214)   SPECIAL CHOCOLATE DREAM BALLS

Preparation Time: 10 minutes + chilling time		Servings: 8

Ingredients:	✓ 1/2 tsp ground cinnamon	Directions:
✓ 3 tbsp cocoa powder	✓ 1/2 cup vegan chocolate, broken into chunks	Add the cocoa powder, dates, tahini and cinnamon to the bowl of your food processor. Process until the mixture forms a ball.
✓ 8 fresh dates, pitted and soaked for 15 minutes	✓ 1 tbsp coconut oil, at room temperature	Use a cookie scoop to portion the mixture into 1-ounce portions. Roll the balls and refrigerate them for at least 30 minutes.
✓ 2 tbsp tahini, at room temperature		Meanwhile, microwave the chocolate until melted; add in the coconut oil and whisk to combine well.
		Dip the chocolate balls in the coating and store them in your refrigerator until ready to serve. Enjoy

215)   EVERYDAY LAST-MINUTE MACAROONS

Preparation Time: 15 minutes		Servings: 10

Ingredients:	✓ 1 tsp ground anise	Directions:
✓ 3 cups coconut flakes, sweetened	✓ 1 tsp vanilla extract	Begin by preheating your oven to 325 degrees F. Line the cookie sheets with parchment paper
✓ 9 ounces canned coconut milk, sweetened		Thoroughly combine all the ingredients until everything is well incorporated.
		Use a cookie scoop to drop mounds of the batter onto the prepared cookie sheets.
		Bake for about 11 minutes until they are lightly browned. Enjoy

216)

216) OLD-FASHIONED RATAFIAS

Preparation Time: 20 minutes		Servings: 8

Ingredients:

- ✓ 2 ounces all-purpose flour
- ✓ 2 ounces almond flour
- ✓ 1 tsp baking powder
- ✓ 2 tbsp applesauce
- ✓ 5 ounces caster sugar
- ✓ 1 ½ ounces vegan butter
- ✓ 4 drops of ratafia essence

Directions:

Start by preheating your oven to 330 degrees F. Line a cookie sheet with parchment paper.

Thoroughly combine all the ingredients until everything is well incorporated.

Use a cookie scoop to drop mounds of the batter onto the prepared cookie sheet.

Bake for about 15 minutes until they are lightly browned. Enjoy

217) ASIAN JASMINE RICE PUDDING WITH DRIED APRICOTS

Preparation Time: 20 minutes		Servings: 4

Ingredients:

- ✓ 1 cup jasmine rice, rinsed
- ✓ 1 cup water
- ✓ 1 cup almond milk
- ✓ 1/2 cup brown sugar
- ✓ A pinch of salt
- ✓ A pinch of grated nutmeg
- ✓ 1/2 cup dried apricots, chopped
- ✓ 1/4 tsp cinnamon powder
- ✓ 1 tsp vanilla extract

Directions:

Add the rice and water to a saucepan. Cover the saucepan and bring the water to a boil.

Turn the heat to low; let it simmer for another 10 minutes until all the water is absorbed.

Then, add in the remaining ingredients and stir to combine. Let it simmer for 10 minutes more or until the pudding has thickened. Enjoy

218) EASY OATMEAL AND PEANUT BUTTER BREAKFAST BAR

Preparation Time: 10 minutes		Servings: 8

Ingredients:

- ✓ 1½ cups date, pit removed
- ✓ ½ cup peanut butter
- ✓ ½ cup old-fashioned rolled oats
- ✓ 1½ cups date, pit removed
- ✓ ½ cup peanut butter
- ✓ ½ cup old-fashioned rolled oats

Directions:

- ❖ Grease and line an 8" x 8" baking tin with parchment and pop to one side.
- ❖ Grab your food processor, add the dates and whizz until chopped.
- ❖ Add the peanut butter and the oats and pulse.
- ❖ Scoop into the baking tin then pop into the fridge or freezer until set.
- ❖ Serve and enjoy.

219) SPECIAL PORRIDGE WITH STRAWBERRIES AND COCONUT

Preparation Time: 12 minutes		Servings: 2

Ingredients:

- ✓ 1 tbsp flax seed powder
- ✓ 1 oz olive oil
- ✓ 1 tbsp coconut flour
- ✓ 1 pinch ground chia seeds
- ✓ 5 tbsp coconut cream
- ✓ Thawed frozen strawberries

Directions:

- ❖ In a small bowl, mix the flax seed powder with the 3 tbsp water, and allow soaking for 5 minutes.
- ❖ Place a non-stick saucepan over low heat and pour in the olive oil, vegan "flax egg," coconut flour, chia seeds, and coconut cream.
- ❖ Cook the mixture while stirring continuously until your desired consistency is achieved. Turn the heat off and spoon the porridge into serving bowls.
- ❖ Top with 4 to 6 strawberries and serve immediately.

220)   CLASSIC BROCCOLI BROWNS

Preparation Time: 35 minutes		Servings: 4

Ingredients:

✓ 3 tbsp flax seed powder
✓ 1 head broccoli, cut into florets
✓ ½ white onion, grated
✓ 1 tsp salt
✓ 1 tbsp freshly ground black pepper
✓ 5 tbsp plant butter, for frying

Directions:

❖ In a small bowl, mix the flax seed powder with 9 tbsp water, and allow soaking for 5 minutes. Pour the broccoli into a food processor and pulse a few times until smoothly grated.

❖ Transfer the broccoli into a bowl, add the vegan "flax egg," white onion, salt, and black pepper. Use a spoon to mix the ingredients evenly and set aside 5 to 10 minutes to firm up a bit. Place a large non-stick skillet over medium heat and drop 1/3 of the plant butter to melt until no longer shimmering.

❖ Ladle scoops of the broccoli mixture into the skillet (about 3 to 4 hash browns per batch). Flatten the pancakes to measure 3 to 4 inches in diameter, and fry until golden brown on one side, 4 minutes. Turn the pancakes with a spatula and cook the other side to brown too, another 5 minutes.

❖ Transfer the hash browns to a serving plate and repeat the frying process for the remaining broccoli mixture. Serve the hash browns warm with green salad.

221)   ITALIAN AVOCADO SANDWICH WITHOUT BREAD

Preparation Time: 10 minutes		Servings: 2

Ingredients:

✓ 1 avocado, sliced
✓ 1 large red tomato, sliced
✓ 2 oz gem lettuce leaves
✓ ½ oz plant butter
✓ 1 oz tofu, sliced
✓ Freshly chopped parsley to garnish

Directions:

❖ Put the avocado on a plate and place the tomato slices by the avocado. Arrange the lettuce (with the inner side facing you) on a flat plate to serve as the base of the sandwich.

❖ To assemble the sandwich, smear each leaf of the lettuce with plant butter, and arrange some tofu slices in the leaves. Then, share the avocado and tomato slices on each cheese. Garnish with parsley and serve.

222) LOVELY TOFU SCRAMBLE

Preparation Time: 46 minutes		Servings: 4

Ingredients:

- ✓ 8 oz water-packed extra firm tofu
- ✓ 2 tbsp plant butter for frying
- ✓ 1 green bell pepper, finely chopped
- ✓ 1 tomato, finely chopped
- ✓ 2 tbsp freshly chopped scallions
- ✓ Salt and black pepper to taste
- ✓ 1 tsp Mexican-style chili powder
- ✓ 3 oz grated plant-based Parmesan

Directions:

- ❖ Place the tofu in between two parchment papers to drain liquid for about 30 minutes.
- ❖ Melt the plant butter in a large non-stick skillet until no longer foaming. Crumble the tofu into the plant butter and fry until golden brown, stirring occasionally, making sure not to break the tofu into tiny pieces. The goal is to have the tofu like scrambled eggs, about 4 to 6 minutes.
- ❖ Stir in the bell pepper, tomato, scallions, and cook until the vegetables are soft, about 4 minutes. Then, season with salt, black pepper, chili powder, and stir in the cheese to incorporate and melt for about 2 minutes. Spoon the scramble into a serving platter and serve warm

223) EASY LEMON AND ALMOND WAFFLES

Preparation Time: 20 minutes		Servings: 4

Ingredients:

- ✓ 2 tbsp flax seed powder
- ✓ 2/3 cup almond flour
- ✓ 2 ½ tsp baking powder
- ✓ A pinch salt
- ✓ 1 ½ cups almond milk
- ✓ 2 tbsp plant butter
- ✓ 1 cup fresh almond butter
- ✓ 2 tbsp pure maple syrup
- ✓ 1 tsp fresh lemon juice

Directions:

- ❖ In a medium bowl, mix the flaxseed powder with 6 tbsp water and allow soaking for 5 minutes. Add the almond flour, baking powder, salt, and almond milk. Mix until well combined. Preheat a waffle iron and brush with some plant butter. Pour in a quarter cup of the batter, close the iron and cook until the waffles are golden and crisp, 2-3 minutes.
- ❖ Transfer the waffles to a plate and make more waffles using the same process and ingredient proportions. In a bowl, mix the almond butter with the maple syrup and lemon juice. Spread the top with the almond-lemon mixture and serve

224) SOUTHERN AMERICAN APPLE COBBLER WITH RASPBERRIES

Preparation Time: 50 minutes		Servings: 4

Ingredients:

- ✓ 3 apples, chopped
- ✓ 2 tbsp pure date sugar
- ✓ 1 cup fresh raspberries
- ✓ 2 tbsp unsalted plant butter
- ✓ ½ cup whole-wheat flour
- ✓ 1 cup toasted rolled oats
- ✓ 2 tbsp pure date sugar
- ✓ 1 tsp cinnamon powder

Directions:

- ❖ Preheat the oven to 350 F and grease a baking dish with some plant butter.
- ❖ Add apples, date sugar, and 3 tbsp of water to a pot. Cook over low heat until the date sugar melts and then mix in the raspberries. Cook until the fruits soften, 10 minutes. Pour and spread the fruit mixture into the baking dish and set aside.
- ❖ In a blender, add the plant butter, flour, oats, date sugar, and cinnamon powder. Pulse a few times until crumbly. Spoon and spread the mixture on the fruit mix until evenly layered. Bake in the oven for 25 to 30 minutes or until golden brown on top. Remove the dessert, allow cooling for 2 minutes, and serve

225) SWEET CHOCOLATE PEPPERMINT MOUSSE

Preparation Time: 10 minutes + chilling time | | **Servings: 4**

Ingredients:

- ✓ ¼ cup Swerve sugar, divided
- ✓ 4 oz cashew cream cheese, softened
- ✓ 3 tbsp cocoa powder
- ✓ ¾ tsp peppermint extract
- ✓ ½ tsp vanilla extract
- ✓ 1/3 cup coconut cream

Directions:

❖ Put 2 tbsp of Swerve sugar, cashew cream cheese, and cocoa powder in a blender. Add the peppermint extract, ¼ cup warm water, and process until smooth. In a bowl, whip vanilla extract, coconut cream, and the remaining Swerve sugar using a whisk. Fetch out 5-6 tbsp for garnishing. Fold in the cocoa mixture until thoroughly combined. Spoon the mousse into serving cups and chill in the fridge for 30 minutes. Garnish with the reserved whipped cream and serve

226) TASTY RASPBERRIES TURMERIC PANNA COTTA

Preparation Time: 10 minutes + chilling time | | **Servings: 6**

Ingredients:

- ✓ ½ tbsp powdered vegetarian gelatin
- ✓ 2 cups coconut cream
- ✓ ¼ tsp vanilla extract
- ✓ 1 pinch turmeric powder
- ✓ 1 tbsp erythritol
- ✓ 1 tbsp chopped toasted pecans
- ✓ 12 fresh raspberries

Directions:

❖ Mix gelatin and ½ tsp water and allow sitting to dissolve. Pour coconut cream, vanilla extract, turmeric, and erythritol into a saucepan and bring to a boil over medium heat, then simmer for 2 minutes. Turn the heat off. Stir in the gelatin until dissolved. Pour the mixture into 6 glasses, cover with plastic wrap, and refrigerate for 2 hours or more. Top with the pecans and raspberries and serve

227) SPRING BANANA PUDDING

Preparation Time: 25 minutes + cooling time | | **Servings:** 4

Ingredients:

- ✓ 1 cup unsweetened almond milk
- ✓ 2 cups cashew cream
- ✓ ¾ cup + 1 tbsp pure date sugar
- ✓ ¼ tsp salt
- ✓ 3 tbsp corn-starch
- ✓ 2 tbsp plant butter, cut into 4 pieces
- ✓ 1 tsp vanilla extract
- ✓ 2 banana, sliced

Directions:

- ❖ In a medium pot, mix almond milk, cashew cream, date sugar, and salt. Cook over medium heat until slightly thickened, 10-15 minutes. Stir in the corn-starch, plant butter, vanilla extract, and banana extract. Cook further for 1 to 2 minutes or until the pudding thickens. Dish the pudding into 4 serving bowls and chill in the refrigerator for at least 1 hour. To serve, top with the bananas and enjoy

228) EVERYDAY BAKED APPLES FILLED WITH NUTS

Preparation Time: 35 minutes + cooling time | | **Servings:** 4

Ingredients:

- ✓ 4 gala apples
- ✓ 3 tbsp pure maple syrup
- ✓ 4 tbsp almond flour
- ✓ 6 tbsp pure date sugar
- ✓ 6 tbsp plant butter, cold and cubed
- ✓ 1 cup chopped mixed nuts

Directions:

- ❖ Preheat the oven the 400 F.
- ❖ Slice off the top of the apples and use a melon baller or spoon to scoop out the cores of the apples. In a bowl, mix the maple syrup, almond flour, date sugar, butter, and nuts. Spoon the mixture into the apples and then bake in the oven for 25 minutes or until the nuts are golden brown on top and the apples soft. Remove the apples from the oven, allow cooling, and serve

229) SUMMER MINT ICE CREAM

Preparation Time: 10 minutes + chilling time | | **Servings:** 4

Ingredients:

- ✓ 2 avocados, pitted
- ✓ 1 ¼ cups coconut cream
- ✓ ½ tsp vanilla extract
- ✓ 2 tbsp erythritol
- ✓ 2 tsp chopped mint leaves

Directions:

- ❖ Into a blender, spoon the avocado pulps, pour in the coconut cream, vanilla extract, erythritol, and mint leaves. Process until smooth. Pour the mixture into your ice cream maker and freeze according to the manufacturer's instructions. When ready, remove and scoop the ice cream into bowls. Serve

230) TASTY CARDAMOM COCONUT FAT BOMBS

Preparation Time: 10 minutes | | **Servings:** 6

Ingredients:

- ✓ ½ cup grated coconut
- ✓ 3 oz plant butter, softened
- ✓ ¼ tsp green cardamom powder
- ✓ ½ tsp vanilla extract
- ✓ ¼ tsp cinnamon powder

Directions:

- ❖ Pour the grated coconut into a skillet and roast until lightly brown. Set aside to cool. In a bowl, combine butter, half of the coconut, cardamom, vanilla, and cinnamon. Form balls from the mixture and roll each one in the remaining coconut. Refrigerate until ready to serve

231)   HUNGARIAN CINNAMON FAUX RICE PUDDING

Preparation Time: 25 minutes		Servings: 6

Ingredients:	✓ 1 cup mashed tofu ✓ 2 oz fresh strawberries	Directions:
✓ 1 ¼ cups coconut cream ✓ 1 tsp vanilla extract ✓ 1 tsp cinnamon powder		❖ Pour the coconut cream into a bowl and whisk until a soft peak forms. Mix in the vanilla and cinnamon. Lightly fold in the vegan cottage cheese and refrigerate for 10 to 15 minutes to set. Spoon into serving glasses, top with the strawberries and serve immediately

232)   SWEET WHITE CHOCOLATE FUDGE

Preparation Time: 20 minutes + chilling time		Servings: 6

Ingredients:	✓ 3 oz vegan white chocolate ✓ Swerve sugar for sprinkling	Directions:
✓ 2 cups coconut cream ✓ 1 tsp vanilla extract ✓ 3 oz plant butter		❖ Pour coconut cream and vanilla into a saucepan and bring to a boil over medium heat, then simmer until reduced by half, 15 minutes. Stir in plant butter until the batter is smooth. Chop white chocolate into bits and stir in the cream until melted. Pour the mixture into a baking sheet; chill in the fridge for 3 hours. Cut into squares, sprinkle with swerve sugar, and serve

233)   ITALIAN MACEDONIA SALAD WITH COCONUT AND PECANS

Preparation Time: 15 minutes + cooling time		Servings: 4

Ingredients:	✓ 4 tbsp toasted pecans, chopped ✓ 1 cup pineapple tidbits, drained ✓ 1 (11-oz) can mandarin oranges ✓ ¾ cup maraschino cherries, stems removed	Directions:
✓ 1 cup pure coconut cream ✓ ½ tsp vanilla extract ✓ 2 bananas, cut into chunks ✓ 1 ½ cups coconut flakes		❖ In a medium bowl, mix the coconut cream and vanilla extract until well combined. ❖ In a larger bowl, combine the bananas, coconut flakes, pecans, pineapple, oranges, and cherries until evenly distributed. Pour on the coconut cream mixture and fold well into the salad. Chill in the refrigerator for 1 hour and serve afterward

234)   AUTHENTIC BERRY HAZELNUT TRIFLE

Preparation Time: 10 minutes		Servings: 4

Ingredients:	✓ 1 tbsp vanilla extract ✓ 3 oz fresh strawberries ✓ 2 oz toasted hazelnuts	Directions:
✓ 1 ½ ripe avocados ✓ ¾ cup coconut cream ✓ Zest and juice of ½ a lemon		❖ In a bowl, add avocado pulp, coconut cream, lemon zest and juice, and half of the vanilla extract. Mix with an immersion blender. Put the strawberries and remaining vanilla in another bowl and use a fork to mash the fruits. In a tall glass, alternate layering the cream and strawberry mixtures. Drop a few hazelnuts on each and serve the dessert immediately

235) VEGETARIAN AVOCADO TRUFFLES WITH CHOCOLATE COATING

Preparation Time: 5 minutes		Servings: 6

Ingredients:

- ✓ 1 ripe avocado, pitted
- ✓ ½ tsp vanilla extract
- ✓ ½ tsp lemon zest
- ✓ 5 oz dairy-free dark chocolate
- ✓ 1 tbsp coconut oil
- ✓ 1 tbsp unsweetened cocoa powder

Directions:

- ❖ Scoop the pulp of the avocado into a bowl and mix with the vanilla using an immersion blender. Stir in the lemon zest and a pinch of salt. Pour the chocolate and coconut oil into a safe microwave bowl and melt in the microwave for 1 minute. Add to the avocado mixture and stir. Allow cooling to firm up a bit. Form balls out of the mix. Roll each ball in the cocoa powder and serve immediately

236) DELICIOUS VANILLA BERRY TARTS

Preparation Time: 35 minutes + cooling time		Servings: 4

Ingredients:

- ✓ 4 tbsp flaxseed powder
- ✓ 1/3 cup whole-wheat flour
- ✓ ½ tsp salt
- ✓ ¼ cup plant butter, crumbled
- ✓ 3 tbsp pure malt syrup
- ✓ 6 oz cashew cream
- ✓ 6 tbsp pure date sugar
- ✓ ¾ tsp vanilla extract
- ✓ 1 cup mixed frozen berries

Directions:

- ❖ Preheat oven to 350 F and grease mini pie pans with cooking spray. In a bowl, mix flaxseed powder with 12 tbsp water and allow soaking for 5 minutes. In a large bowl, combine flour and salt. Add in butter and whisk until crumbly. Pour in the vegan "flax egg" and malt syrup and mix until smooth dough forms. Flatten the dough on a flat surface, cover with plastic wrap, and refrigerate for 1 hour.
- ❖ Dust a working surface with some flour, remove the dough onto the surface, and using a rolling pin, flatten the dough to a 1-inch diameter circle. Use a large cookie cutter, cut out rounds of the dough and fit into the pie pans. Use a knife to trim the edges of the pan. Lay a parchment paper on the dough cups, pour on some baking beans, and bake in the oven until golden brown, 15-20 minutes. Remove the pans from the oven, pour out the baking beans, and allow cooling. In a bowl, mix cashew cream, date sugar, and vanilla extract. Divide the mixture into the tart cups and top with berries. Serve

237) BEST HOMEMADE CHOCOLATES WITH COCONUT AND RAISINS

Preparation Time: 10 minutes + chilling time		Servings: 20

Ingredients:

- ✓ 1/2 cup cacao butter, melted
- ✓ 1/3 cup peanut butter
- ✓ 1/4 cup agave syrup
- ✓ A pinch of grated nutmeg
- ✓ A pinch of coarse salt
- ✓ 1/2 tsp vanilla extract
- ✓ 1 cup dried coconut, shredded
- ✓ 6 ounces dark chocolate, chopped
- ✓ 3 ounces raisins

Directions:

- ❖ Thoroughly combine all the ingredients, except for the chocolate, in a mixing bowl.
- ❖ Spoon the mixture into molds. Leave to set hard in a cool place.
- ❖ Melt the dark chocolate in your microwave. Pour in the melted chocolate until the fillings are covered. Leave to set hard in a cool place.
- ❖ Enjoy

238) SIMPLE MOCHA FUDGE

Preparation Time: 1 hour 10 minutes		Servings: 20

Ingredients:

- ✓ 1 cup cookies, crushed
- ✓ 1/2 cup almond butter
- ✓ 1/4 cup agave nectar
- ✓ 6 ounces dark chocolate, broken into chunks
- ✓ 1 tsp instant coffee
- ✓ A pinch of grated nutmeg
- ✓ A pinch of salt

Directions:

- ❖ Line a large baking sheet with parchment paper.
- ❖ Melt the chocolate in your microwave and add in the remaining ingredients; stir to combine well.
- ❖ Scrape the batter into a parchment-lined baking sheet. Place it in your freezer for at least 1 hour to set.
- ❖ Cut into squares and serve. Enjoy

239) EAST ALMOND AND CHOCOLATE CHIP BARS

Preparation Time: 40 minutes		**Servings: 10**

Ingredients:

- ✓ 1/2 cup almond butter
- ✓ 1/4 cup coconut oil, melted
- ✓ 1/4 cup agave syrup
- ✓ 1 tsp vanilla extract
- ✓ 1/4 tsp sea salt
- ✓ 1/4 tsp grated nutmeg
- ✓ 1/2 tsp ground cinnamon
- ✓ 2 cups almond flour
- ✓ 1/4 cup flaxseed meal
- ✓ 1 cup vegan chocolate, cut into chunks
- ✓ 1 1/3 cups almonds, ground
- ✓ 2 tbsp cacao powder
- ✓ 1/4 cup agave syrup

Directions:

- ❖ In a mixing bowl, thoroughly combine the almond butter, coconut oil, 1/4 cup of agave syrup, vanilla, salt, nutmeg and cinnamon.
- ❖ Gradually stir in the almond flour and flaxseed meal and stir to combine. Add in the chocolate chunks and stir again.
- ❖ In a small mixing bowl, combine the almonds, cacao powder and agave syrup. Now, spread the ganache onto the cake. Freeze for about 30 minutes, cut into bars and serve well chilled. Enjoy

240) ALMOND BUTTER COOKIES

Preparation Time: 45 minutes		**Servings: 10**

Ingredients:

- ✓ 3/4 cup all-purpose flour
- ✓ 1/2 tsp baking soda
- ✓ 1/4 tsp kosher salt
- ✓ 1 flax egg
- ✓ 1/4 cup coconut oil, at room temperature
- ✓ 2 tbsp almond milk
- ✓ 1/2 cup brown sugar
- ✓ 1/2 cup almond butter
- ✓ 1/2 tsp ground cinnamon
- ✓ 1/2 tsp vanilla

Directions:

- ❖ In a mixing bowl, combine the flour, baking soda and salt.
- ❖ In another bowl, combine the flax egg, coconut oil, almond milk, sugar, almond butter, cinnamon and vanilla. Stir the wet mixture into the dry ingredients and stir until well combined.
- ❖ Place the batter in your refrigerator for about 30 minutes. Shape the batter into small cookies and arrange them on a parchment-lined cookie pan.
- ❖ Bake in the preheated oven at 350 degrees F for approximately 12 minutes. Transfer the pan to a wire rack to cool at room temperature. Enjoy

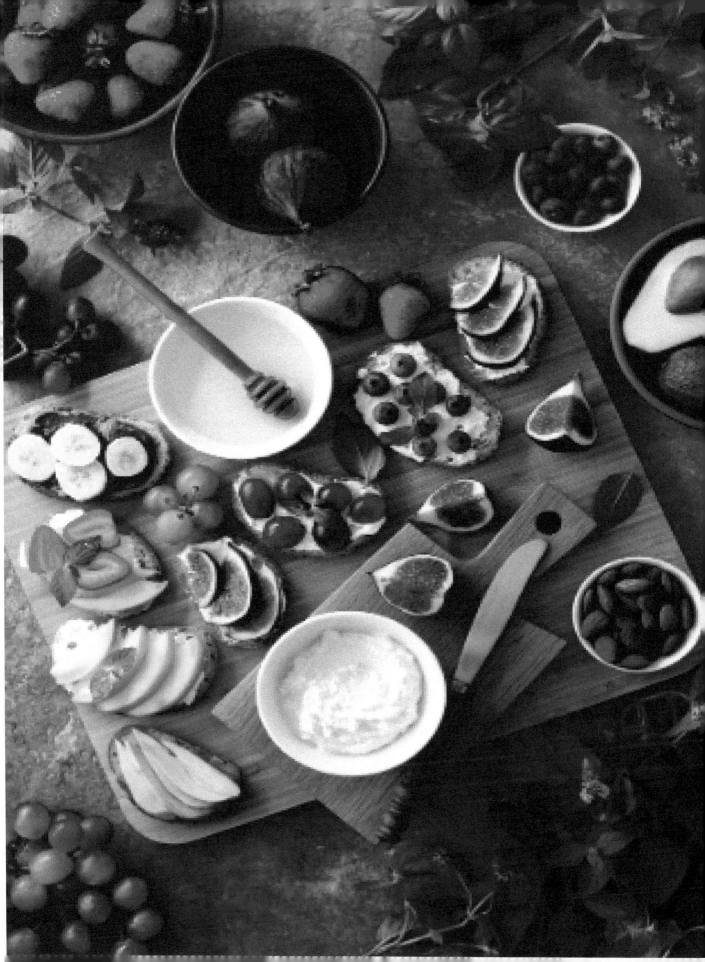

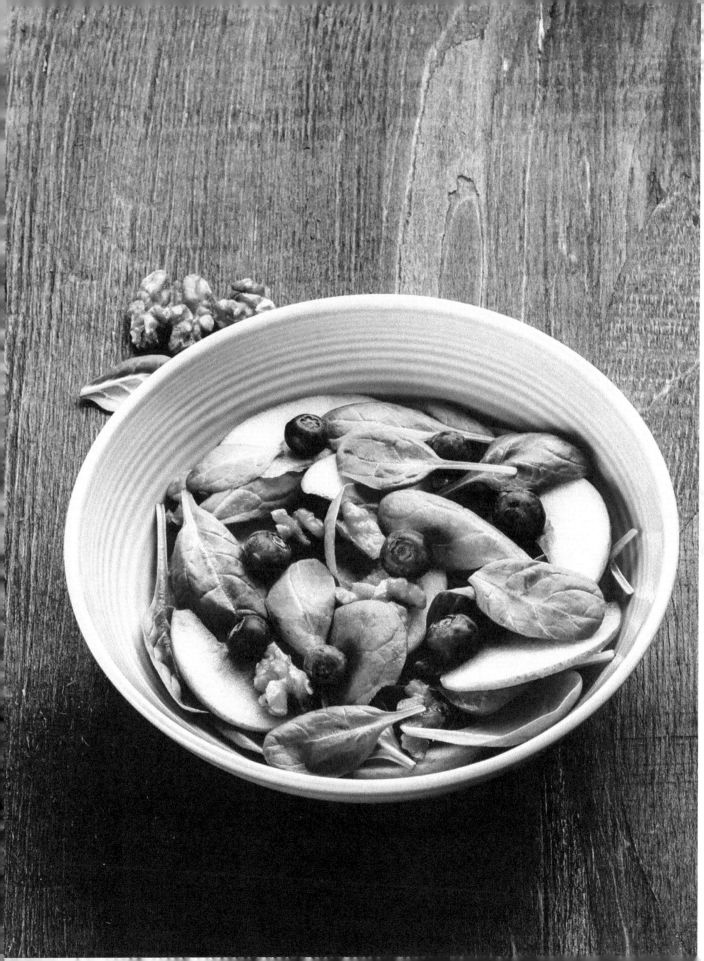

Bibliography

FROM THE SAME AUTHOR

PLANT-BASED DIET FOR MEN Cookbook - The Best 120+ High-Protein Green Meals! Make your body STRONG and FIT with the Healthiest Recipes for Him!

PLANT-BASED DIET FOR WOMEN Cookbook - More than 120 High-Protein Recipes to stay TONE and have more ENERGY! Start your Green Lifestyle with one of the Healthiest Diet for Her Overall!

PLANT-BASED DIET Cookbook - The Best 120+ Green Recipes for a healthier Lifestyle! Stay FIT and have more ENERGY with many High-Protein Vegan and Vegetarian Meals!

PLANT-BASED COOKBOOK FOR STUDENTS - FOCUS ON STUDYING - The Best 120+ Recipes to stay more CONCENTRATED and have more ENERGY! Maintain Perfect your Focus on Studying with many High-Protein Vegan and Vegetarian Meals!

PLANT-BASED DIET FOR COUPLE Cookbook - More than 220 High-Protein Vegetarian Recipes to Surprise your Partner in the Kitchen! Start your Healthier Lifestyle with the Best Green Meals to Make Together!

HIGH PROTEIN PLANT-BASED COOKBOOK FOR ATHLETES - Many High-Protein Vegan and Vegetarian Recipes to Boost your Body to the TOP! The Best 220+ Green and Healthy Recipes to Perform your Muscles and Sculpt your Abs stay LIGHT!

PLANT-BASED DIET FOR HEALTHY MUM & KIDS Cookbook - The Best 220+ Green Recipes to make with your Kids! Start a HAPPY and HEALTHY Lifestyle with the Quickest Vegetarian and Vegan Recipes for your Family!

QUICK AND EASY PLANT-BASED DIET Cookbook - The Simplest and Quickest High-Protein Green Recipes to Start Your Healthy Lifestyle! Stay LIGHT cooking More Than 220+ Very Easy Meals Without Stress!

PLANT-BASED DIET FOR FITNESS WOMAN Cookbook - More than 220 Super Healthy Vegan and Vegetarian Recipes to Increase your Energy, Detox Your Body, and Improve your Body Tone to the TOP! Stay FIT and LIGHT with these Best Selected High-Protein Green Meals!

PLANT-BASED FOR YOUNG ATHLETES Cookbook - Many Green and Healthy Recipes to Perform your Body Tone while stay LIGHT! The Best 220+ High-Protein Vegetarian Recipes to stay Fit and Start a New Lifestyle!

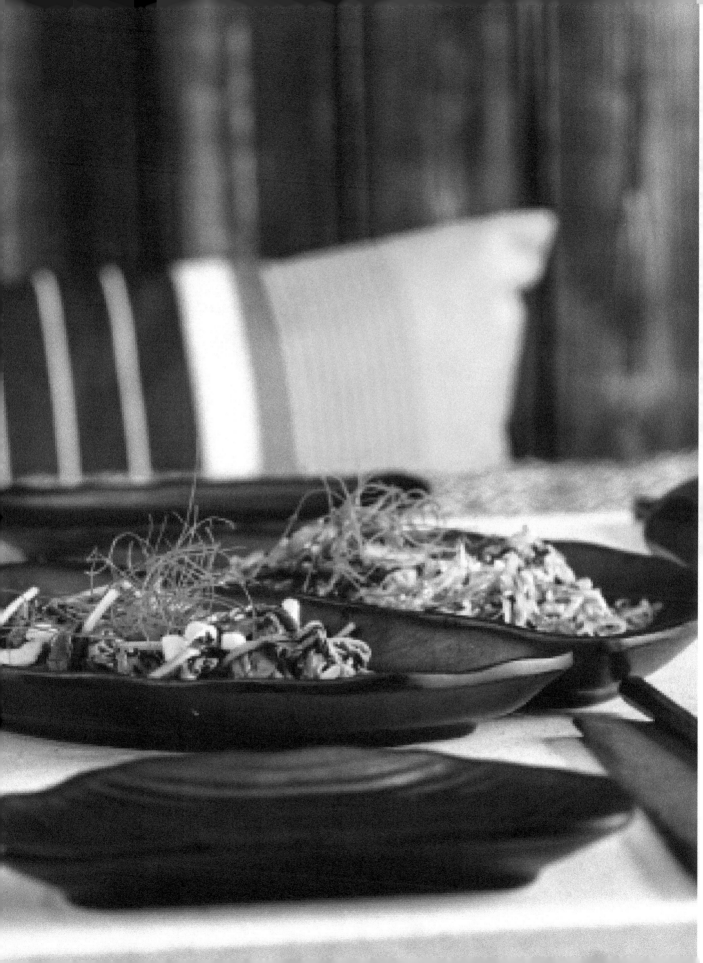

Conclusion

Thanks for reading "The Plant-Based Diet for Couple *Cookbook*"

Follow the right habits it is essential to have a healthy Lifestyle, and the Plant-Based diet is the best solution!

I hope you liked this Cookbook!

I wish you to achieve all your goal!

William Miller

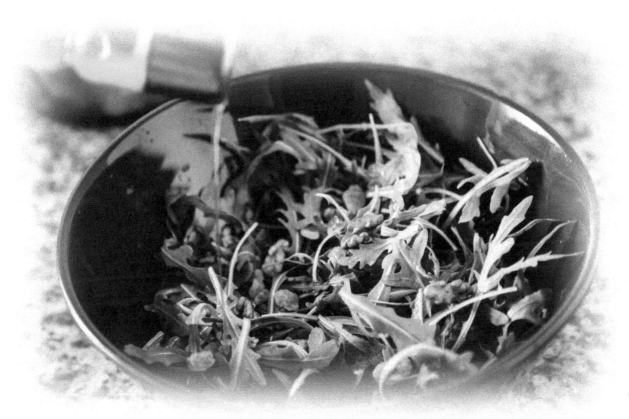

9 781803 119236